# PAYING PHYSICIANS

## Options for Controlling Cost, Volume, and Intensity of Services

# PAYING PHYSICIANS
## Options for Controlling Cost, Volume, and Intensity of Services

Mark V. Pauly

John M. Eisenberg

Margaret Higgins Radany

M. Haim Erder

Roger Feldman

J. Sanford Schwartz

Health Administration Press
Ann Arbor, Michigan    1992

96  95  94  93  92      5  4  3  2  1


**Library of Congress Cataloging-in-Publication Data**

Paying physicians : options for controlling cost, volume, and intensity of services / Mark V. Pauly . . . [et al.].
   p.    cm.
  Includes bibliographical references and index.
  ISBN 0-910701-87-3 (alk. paper : softbound)
  1. Medicare.  2. Medical fees.  3. Physicians—United States—Supply and demand.  I. Pauly, Mark V., date.
  [DNLM:  1. Delivery of Health Care—economics—United States.
2. Fees, Medical—United States.  3. Medicare—economics.  4. Physicians—psychology—United States.  W 84 AA1 P297]
RA412.5.U6P39    1992    338.4'33621'0973—dc20
DNLM/DLC for Library of Congress    92-1567 CIP

The paper used in this publication meets the minimum requirements of American National Standard for Information Sciences—Permanence of Paper for Printed Library Materials, ANSI Z39.48-1984.  ∞ ™

Health Administration Press
A division of the Foundation of the
  American College of Healthcare Executives
1021 East Huron Street
Ann Arbor, Michigan 48104-9990
(313) 764-1380

# Contents

# Acknowledgments

The genesis of this book was a research project the authors first performed for the Health Care Financing Administration before the present reforms in Medicare physician payment were implemented. In 1988, HCFA requested a "thoughtful analysis" of various approaches to controlling the volume and intensity of physician services, concerned that the impending implementation of a fee schedule in Medicare might do little in and of itself to control aggregate expenditures. The immediate result of our project was an over-budget, oversized report, *Issues Related to the Volume and Intensity of Physician Services*, that indicated the complexity of this subject and the interest we had in analyzing it. The first acknowledgment must therefore go to the Health Care Financing Administration for funding this initial effort.

While we were working on this project, the American Medical Association was also following the issue of Medicare payment reform closely; our mutual interest in the subject of volume controls resulted in a small conference hosted jointly by the American Medical Association and the University of Pennsylvania's Leonard Davis Institute of Health Economics (where our study was based). Approximately 25 health economists, physicians, policy analysts, and researchers convened to focus on three papers related to volume control in the Medicare program and discuss related issues. These papers, cited heavily in the first three chapters of this book, are one by Patrick S. Cotter on the history, performance, and evaluation of physician service coverage under Medicare; a second by Kathryn Langwell and Gene Falk on a framework for analysis of the growth in volume of physician services; and a third by Gerard J. Wedig on the trends in Medicare Part B spending prior to and following the fee freeze of the mid-1980s. These authors in particular, and all who participated in the conference, helped us to shape and refine our thinking on many of the issues discussed here.

Finally, we are indebted to Jennifer Conway of the Leonard Davis Institute of Health Economics for her invaluable editorial and organizational assistance, and to Traci Frank and Martha Beale for their expert and tireless word processing of the manuscript for this book.

Part I

# Background and Theory

# Chapter 1

# Issues in Physician Payment:
# An Introduction and Overview

Controlling the volume and intensity of physician services has been, and will probably remain, a primary tactic in the ongoing battle to contain health care costs in the United States. Over the past two decades, changes in the volume and intensity of care have accounted for more than half of the real growth in physician spending. In 1989, federal policymakers followed several years of piecemeal efforts to control physician payment with the enactment of significant changes in Medicare's supplementary medical insurance (SMI) program, the part of Medicare that pays for physician services. Guided by three objectives—to rationalize physician payment, to control Medicare program costs, and to maintain beneficiary access to high-quality medical care—this package represents focused reform of Medicare Part B, as SMI is commonly known (PPRC 1990). The resulting changes, scheduled to be implemented over a four-year period beginning in 1992, promise to stimulate new approaches to physician payment in the private sector and to unleash substantial repercussions throughout the health care industry.

The first component of the three-part Medicare Part B restructuring is a major change in the method of physician payment: a predetermined schedule of fees will be used, based on the relative values of various services and adjusted for the geographic location of the physician. The fees will be uniform for all physicians, regardless of their specialty or prior charges. The second component is the implementation of controls to keep the overall volume of services provided to Medicare recipients from growing more rapidly than Congress desires. The third reform involves setting strict limits on the extent to which physicians can bill Medicare beneficiaries for charges in excess of what Medicare will pay.

Medicare's new method of physician payment, the fee schedule, was designed to replace the "customary, prevailing, and reasonable" (CPR) approach that has been the health insurance industry's payment standard for 30 years. The CPR payment approach is based on the historical charges of the individual physician as well as those of his or her colleagues in the same specialty and geographic area. Payment for a specific service is determined by the lowest of the actual charge, the physician's customary charge for that service, or the prevailing charge (comparable physicians' prior billings for that service). In the Medicare program, increases in prevailing charges have been limited since 1976 to increases in the Medicare economic index (MEI), which measures changes in practice expenses and general earnings (OTA 1986).

The CPR system has had a number of problems. Some analysts argue that it has been inherently inflationary. If a physician's customary charge were lower than the prevailing charge, that physician might be paid less by Medicare than other physicians would be paid for the same service. The CPR scheme has encouraged such a physician to increase his or her charges in one year in order to set the base for higher actual payments in subsequent years (Holahan, Hadley, and Scanlon 1979; Langwell and Nelson 1986; Wilensky and Rossiter 1986). With price increases limited by the MEI, however, the incentive to raise fees disappears. The CPR payment approach also allegedly has induced physicians to provide certain services rather than others because of reimbursement incentives, with prices for the performance of specific procedures being generally higher, considering the physician time required, than those for the evaluation and nonprocedural management of disease. Finally, CPR payment has led to interregional differences in allowed fees that cannot be explained completely by differences in the cost of nonphysician inputs for providing care (Lee et al. 1990; Levy et al. 1990).

Although Medicare's new fee schedule will continue the fee-for-service basis for Medicare payment, it is intended to address the inflationary incentives of the CPR approach for some physicians by removing the dependence of current-period reimbursement on prior-period charges. The fee schedule is based on assigned values, in relative terms, for the various services physicians can provide. These values take into consideration such factors as the physician's time and effort, practice expenses, and the cost of malpractice insurance (PPRC 1990; Ginsburg, LeRoy, and Hammons 1990; Iglehart 1990; Lee et al. 1990). Accordingly, this specific fee schedule is referred to as a *resource-based relative value scale* (RBRVS). Assigning relative values in this way is expected to rationalize prices and thereby remove the supposed incentives for the provision of procedural services.

To arrive at an actual fee for each service, the relative value is multiplied by a dollar conversion factor. In the Medicare program, fees are then to be adjusted for geographic location to account for differences across localities, both in practice expenses (the prices physicians have to pay for things such as wages, supplies, and rent) and in living expenses. The result of these computations is the *Medicare fee schedule* (MFS). Yearly changes in Medicare's dollar conversion factor are to be based on the rate of general inflation and, as will be described shortly, congressional preferences about the volume of services provided. Fee updates will not be based on any individual physician's charges, thereby eliminating one of the inflationary aspects of the initial phases of the CPR system, that is, the incentive to increase fees continually.

Under the new structure, the volume (i.e., the actual aggregate number) of Medicare services is to be controlled by the use of a volume performance standard. Each year, Congress must consider recommendations from the Physician Payment Review Commission and the Department of Health and Human Services, and determine the "appropriate" or desired increase in expenditures for Medicare physician services. Imposing such standards on overall spending will, of course, affect the intensity of care (i.e., the number and combination of services provided to individual patients) as well as the volume. When setting this volume performance standard, Congress will consider general inflation, the number of Medicare beneficiaries, changes in technology, and evidence of inadequate access to care and inappropriate use of services for the Medicare population (PPRC 1990). Ultimately, the choice will be political. Actual increases in expenditures will then be monitored against this standard. If expenditures are excessive, relative to the congressional standard, in any given year the update in the fee schedule's dollar conversion factor will be reduced (PPRC 1990; Ginsburg et al. 1990; Iglehart 1990; Lee et al. 1990). The purpose of linking volume and price is twofold: it is intended to control aggregate spending and to discourage (through the penalty of lower prices) the provision of services that Congress is unwilling to support.

The plan for maintaining beneficiary access to care is to provide financial protection for Medicare beneficiaries by limiting balance billing, the amount physicians are permitted to receive from patients in excess of the amount Medicare will pay. The premiums that the elderly pay to participate in Part B increased by 38.5 percent in 1988 and 12.5 percent in 1989 (Holahan, Dor, and Zuckerman 1990), which fueled congressional concern about the financial liability of beneficiaries. This reform, scheduled to be phased in by 1993, will prohibit physicians from charging more than 115 percent of the Medicare fee level. This approach will replace the complex system of maximum allowable actual charge limits, which dictates allowable charges based on individual physicians' charges in relation to the relevant prevailing charge (PPRC 1990).

The consequences of the changes in Medicare Part B are expected to be considerable throughout both the public and the private health care systems. It is hoped, for example, that the move to the RBRVS will modify the very practice of medicine through the use of economic incentives to produce a more desirable mix of services. Significant reallocations of income among physician specialties, in what some hope will be a more equitable fashion, are expected as a result.

The implementation of controls on the volume of physician services is even more revolutionary. It indicates that Congress hopes to achieve cost containment by doing more than simply constraining all fees (PPRC 1990; Iglehart 1990). To a degree not seen previously, physicians themselves will now be responsible for rationing Medicare dollars, and they will operate under the specter of financial penalty if they are not successful.

Likewise, limits on balance billing will be more severe than ever before. Some physicians may respond by avoiding Medicare patients. Such action, especially in combination with the other effects noted above, would reduce the Medicare beneficiary's access to care and could affect the prices faced by private patients and their insurance companies.

Despite (or perhaps because of) the passage of the RBRVS legislation, active debate continues on how to implement the broad contours of a fee-schedule approach. As the Medicare reforms are implemented, there exists the opportunity to alter or refine the details of the program. How a fee schedule ultimately works, and what additional alterations in payment arrangements might make sense, are issues that are still unsettled. Evaluation of the likely effects of a fee schedule and consideration of additional means to achieve the policy's desired results are thus important contributors to the long-range effectiveness of these Medicare reforms and similar private-sector efforts.

## What This Book Is About

As the Medicare Part B reforms indicate, a major health care cost-containment strategy is to change physician behavior by imposing limits on the volume and intensity of the services that physicians provide. Further legislative or private-sector attempts to influence medical practice in this way are likely. The consequences of such policies are uncertain, however, given the complexity of the health care market, the unpredictability of physician behavior in response to financial incentives, and the ever-changing technology of medicine.

In this book, empirical clues and economic and behavioral theory form the basis for a sketch of some of the scenarios that are likely to occur for Medicare beneficiaries and throughout the health care system as a result of the current and potential changes in physician payment methods. The main focus of the book is on the impact of various methods that could be used to control the volume of physician services. The effects of the change from a charge-based payment system to a resource-based system are also addressed. Although the analyses herein are generally oriented toward the effect of changes in the Medicare program, many of the same issues hold for private insurers (at least for large ones), so private-sector concerns have been discussed whenever possible. The book also covers the likely impact of other strategies that could be used to achieve the same goals. To illustrate the context within which the present reforms have occurred, Chapter 2 highlights the pertinent history of the Medicare Part B program. An awareness of the magnitude of Part B expenditure increases over the years and the history of previous cost-containment efforts provides a basis for understanding the need for and shape of the present reforms. Results of recent research on the factors driving these outpatient and physician costs are also included to illustrate the present emphasis on control of the volume and intensity of physician services.

Several different but plausible theories or models of physician behavior are developed in Chapter 3, and in later chapters an attempt is made to determine how each of these models might respond under each of the policies examined. Because none of the models has proved to be the single best description of physician behavior, all are used to explore the range of possible effects of the Part B reforms. Readers may attach higher subjective probabilities to some of the models than to the others. Tracking each model's predictions through the various policies will not only provide a full catalog of probable policy responses, it will also provide a list that is highly consistent because it is based on a common set of assumptions about physician behavior.

The aims of this book are to alert readers to the range of possible consequences of the physician payment system, to urge them to consider which changes are likely to be most effective (or most beneficial), and thereby to facilitate the development of thoughtful policies by both public and private insurers. To meet these objectives, we raise and address two major questions: What do theory and evidence suggest about the possible effects of various controls on the volume, intensity, and cost of physician services? And what will the effects of the change to a resource-based fee schedule with volume limits be on Medicare beneficiaries and on persons covered by private insurance?

# Possible Effects of Various Controls on the Volume, Intensity, and Cost of Physician Services

## Models of physician behavior

The basis for speculating about the possible effects of controls on physician services is behavioral theory about how physicians respond to the controls and prices they receive. Three models dominate the thinking in this area: the patient agency model, the profit maximization model, and the target-income model. Each is discussed in detail in Chapter 3.

The *profit maximization model* describes a world in which doctors always seek to maximize income net of both practice costs and the cost of their time by providing the greatest number of profitable services that the market will accept. This model recognizes that physicians, like most people, work to make a living, and that they understandably experience some level of concern about their incomes. Because there appears to be considerable latitude in determining what constitutes appropriate care, some physicians may, within perfectly acceptable standards of practice, provide patients with the most and the best care in a way that maximizes their (the physicians') net income.

Physicians may attempt to moderate concern about their own incomes by having a target income in mind that prods them sometimes to provide a more extravagant service than might be absolutely necessary but that still is within the bounds of medical acceptability, given the standards of practice. Under the *target-income model*, if a decrease in price for a given intervention affects a doctor's income significantly, he or she may simply use that or some other intervention more often (if possible) so as to maintain a given income level, or may provide a more profitable one that accomplishes the same thing. The physician can still maintain the desired income by sacrificing a modest amount of the patient's interest, at the margin, especially if the care does no overt harm.

In the *patient agency model*, the net financial rewards of practice are secondary to physicians' concerns about providing the most appropriate care to their patients, the care that balances the benefits of services against any user price the patient pays. Physicians in this model are indifferent to the prices they receive, and changes in their payment simply will not affect their practice as long as such changes do not affect the amount patients pay.

In reality, physician behavior in response to price changes is surely more complex—and more variable—than these simple models would suggest. The behavior of a given physician may change over time or with varying situations, and undoubtedly, considerable differences exist among physicians depending on specialty, location, practice setting, and many other factors. Considering these "pure" models, however, helps to identify the most extreme effects possible, in the aggregate, of a major policy change such as is anticipated in Medicare. Exploring these extreme scenarios of the effect of payment reform and giving thoughtful consideration to the theories themselves (as well as to whatever empirical evidence is available) allows each reader to make a "best guess" about what is most likely to result from various approaches to controlling the volume and intensity of physician services.

**Possible controls on the volume and intensity of physician services**

After reviewing these behavioral theories in Chapter 3, we consider in Part II the possible effects of a variety of potential controls on physician services. Although Congress chose to use a relative value fee schedule along with volume performance standards to address the cost and equity concerns of Medicare, many other mechanisms could have been (and could yet be) implemented in the Medicare program. Likewise, private insurers are searching for ways to control their own spending on physician services and could choose from a range of controls.

We have chosen in this book to consider seven possible approaches to controlling the volume and intensity of physician services. We begin in Chapter 4 with the one that has been used the longest and thus has the greatest empirical evidence of effectiveness: beneficiary copayment. Requiring insured persons to pay some portion of physician charges out of their own pockets as a means of limiting the quantity of care demanded has been a standard approach in Medicare and private indemnity insurance plans. Copayments typically consist of two parts: a fixed deductible, which beneficiaries must pay before the insurance plan pays anything, and coinsurance, a percentage of physician charges beyond the deductible. In addition to reviewing the data on and factors influencing the effectiveness of copayments in limiting the volume and intensity of care, we suggest some changes that might enhance the usefulness of this approach, especially in the Medicare program.

In Chapter 5, we consider as a volume control the simple dissemination of clinical guidelines, accompanied by efforts to educate physicians about the content of the guidelines. Like copayment, guidelines have been used fairly extensively in medicine, and some evidence suggests that they can change practice patterns when developed and disseminated in certain ways. Unlike copayment, however, guidelines have only recently been viewed as a way to control services and expenditures. More often they have been used to inform physicians of appropriate or ideal practice in various clinical situations. After considering the factors that have been shown to influence the utility of guidelines in their more typical use and their likely impacts as volume controls under the various models of physician behavior, we propose some specific approaches to volume and intensity control through the use of clinical guidelines.

Chapter 6 focuses on a control mechanism that, in its multiple forms, has recently become one of the most popular approaches to limiting the volume of services: utilization review. The use of utilization review along with copayment, in both Medicare and private indemnity plans, became widespread in the United States in the 1970s and 1980s, promising to contain health care costs by requiring second opinions for elective surgeries, by reviewing the physician's care either before, after, or during treatment, and by enforcing appropriate care through denial of payment for services deemed unnecessary. We consider the evidence on the effectiveness of these devices and describe some implications based on theory to fill in the empirical blanks.

In Chapter 7 we consider capitation, another approach that has grown in use over the past two decades. By paying a predetermined amount for all health care to be provided to each insured person over a given period, capitation is designed to limit volume and costs by removing the "extra pay for extra services" incentive of fee-for-service payment. Medicare beneficiaries have been allowed to enroll in capitated plans since 1982, with the advantages of lower copayments and perhaps a greater range of benefits. Only 3 percent of Medicare beneficiaries have selected this option, however (PPRC 1988; HCFA 1990). We examine the evidence and offer some thoughts on why capitation may have been less effective than expected.

The focus of Chapter 8 is on a control that will soon be used for the first time in this country: an expenditure target scheme. Expenditure targets are included in the Medicare physician payment changes in the form of volume performance standards, and they are a particularly intriguing type of control. By setting a yearly target for overall expenditure increases, actual spending growth can be monitored against what is thought to be appropriate or ideal. When spending is higher than the targeted amount, prices are adjusted downward (or not increased as much as they might otherwise be) to keep aggregate expenditures within the target. Similar mechanisms have been used with some apparent success in other countries (notably Germany and Canada), and our analysis suggests that expenditure targets have the potential to control costs in the United States as well. Some of the drawbacks of such an approach could be serious, however, and careful monitoring would be needed to detect and, if possible, address them. The chapter includes some thoughts on how this could be done best.

The two final controls we consider, service bundling (Chapter 9) and collapsed procedure codes (Chapter 10), have not been used extensively to date. There has been some use of service bundling in the United States in the form of "global" payments for surgical services, wherein the surgeon's pre- and postoperative care is included in the payment for the surgical procedure itself. Recent legislation has eliminated Medicare payment for most electrocardiogram interpretations on the rationale that such a service should be considered part of the physician visit (AMA 1991). The Canadian province of Quebec has used a similar bundling approach since 1976, with 26 diagnostic and therapeutic procedures bundled together with an office visit so that one fee covers all (Evans et al. 1989).

This approach to payment could be extended in a number of ways; for example, by paying for all care provided during the course of a specific illness, or for all tests, visits, and prescriptions surrounding a major procedure. The notion is that such a payment arrangement, which can be thought of as a kind of partial capitation, would limit volume by discouraging the use of marginally useful services. We consider the various forms this payment scheme could take and the likelihood of its producing significant savings in the long run.

Finally, collapsed procedure codes are intended to address the influence that billing codes have on the choice of and charges for certain services. Multiple procedure codes presently exist for some types of services so that varying levels of intensity—and varying charges—can be indicated on billing forms. Office visits, for example, can be brief, limited, intermediate, extended, or comprehensive, and with each increment in complexity comes an increment in the charge. Collapsing these codes so that there is only one payment for an office visit would, the argument goes, remove incentives to provide a more intense service than is necessary, or to bill for a more intense service than was actually provided. Because no clear definitions exist for most of the "finer" procedure codes, extensive miscoding, either honest or fraudulent, may well occur. Would collapsed codes serve to limit the volume of services provided? With little empirical evidence to go on, we turn to the behavioral theories to examine this question.

Evidence on the extent to which these various controls are currently used is presented in Appendix A at the end of the book. Surveys of Medicare carriers and a sample of private insurers provide an overview of the extent to which volume control is viewed as a viable cost-containment strategy and of the forms it presently takes.

# Effects of the RBRVS with Volume Limits on Medicare and Private Insurance Beneficiaries

As already noted, the changes in Medicare Part B are expected to have widespread effects throughout the health care industry, influencing the costs, processes, and possibly the outcomes of care. Medicare beneficiaries themselves will certainly be affected, but perhaps not always in the positive ways anticipated. At the same time, privately insured patients will undoubtedly experience indirect effects as a variety of forces and counterforces come into play with private insurers responding to the Medicare changes. Part III turns to the potential impact of the resource-based relative value scale with controls on volume and limits on balance billing. Chapter 11 discusses the expected benefits as well as possible negative effects for Medicare beneficiaries, and Chapter 12 looks at the potential effects on the private sector.

## Effects on Medicare beneficiaries

Medicare beneficiaries are expected to benefit from the physician payment changes in a number of ways. First, the change in physician incentives that should follow the change in prices is supposed to induce a greater supply of what is thought to be more appropriate care (and, presumably, better outcomes) for beneficiaries, both in the short run and over time. Supporters of this policy assume that price does influence physician behavior and that its direction is predictable. More generous payments for the provision of so-called evaluation and management services specified by RBRVS are expected to increase the volume of these services. If this happens, Medicare beneficiaries would receive more primary care, with attention given to prevention, counseling, diagnostic workups, and close monitoring of disease. Over the long term, it is argued, the physician specialties in which these services have typically been provided (family practice and internal medicine) will become more rewarding financially, thereby attracting more recruits and improving beneficiaries' access to such care.

At the same time that increasing amounts of such care are anticipated from RBRVS, lower volumes of other kinds of services are expected for those services whose prices are cut. This will yield a benefit if the net effect is more appropriate care. Recent studies have suggested that substantial proportions of many technical procedures are used inappropriately, including common procedures and surgeries such as coronary angiography, coronary artery surgery, endoscopies, and carotid endarterectomy (Chassin et al. 1986; Chassin et al. 1987; Kahn et al. 1988;

Winslow et al. 1988). Because some of the invasive procedures carry significant risks, reduction in the number of unnecessary ones—if that can be accomplished without affecting those that are necessary—will result in an overall improvement in the quality of care.

Another anticipated benefit is the ultimate cost-moderating effect the reforms should have, and the resulting financial advantages for the elderly. In the near term, any savings in program costs attributable to the volume controls and changes in payment method are expected to translate into limited or no increases in Medicare Part B premiums. Perhaps more importantly, in the long run these volume controls may well enable the Medicare program to continue providing the broad coverage and attendant financial security that beneficiaries have come to expect. The other component of the Medicare reforms, limits on balance billing, will further protect the elderly from the expenses associated with illness. Continued financial access to high-quality care is an objective of the present reforms, but such access may not be compatible with lower costs, because lower prices themselves may affect what physicians are willing to supply.

Will the expected benefits be realized? Given the restrictions presented by these reforms, will physicians still be willing to care for Medicare patients? How will privately insured patients and their insurers be affected? These and other concerns are addressed in Chapter 12.

## Impact on the private sector

In a less direct fashion, persons covered by private insurance may also face significant modifications in coverage or care as a result of these Medicare changes. Like the government, private insurers have faced rising expenditures on physician services and have sought to limit them by a number of means. Thus, private insurers will surely be watching these Medicare effects with keen interest and an eye toward using similar controls in their own plans.

There will be other concerns in the private health insurance industry, however. Given the uncertainty about the response of physicians to the Medicare reimbursement changes and limits, private insurers will face difficult decisions. Should they pay higher charges than Medicare, even if it means higher premiums, in order to lure patients who will be attracted by the implicitly greater access to care and physicians, and who are disgruntled with the constraints of the Medicare program? Or should they attempt to limit reimbursements (and premiums) at a lower level and hope they can offer a competitive level of quality at that price?

Although it is not possible to identify the best approach without some knowledge of the actual degree to which the Medicare changes will affect charges to privately insured patients, various strategies can be considered. Certain efforts related to balance billing, volume monitoring, and preferred providers may be useful to private insurers, especially in the uncertain early stages of the Medicare reforms. Perhaps the best private-sector strategy, however, will be to wait and see what happens before changing anything. In Chapter 12, we discuss these various approaches and provide a rationale for watchful waiting.

## A Final Word

The conclusions presented throughout this book may seem frustratingly ambiguous. There is no consensus about which behavioral model best describes reality, and the economic workings of the health care system are far from clear. We therefore cannot say with certainty which approach to the control of physicians' services would be best. What we can do, however, is provide a thoughtful analysis of the relevant issues, pointing out along the way what is and is not known. We can indicate which assumptions about physician behavior make particular predictions a good bet. Our hope is that such an exercise will not only provide practical and immediate guidance for policymaking in an uncertain world but will also plant the seeds for fruitful research, so that future actions can be better informed. We can, in addition, identify worst case scenarios, and try to anticipate them, watch for them, and think about strategies to avert them.

## References

American Medical Association (AMA). 1991. "New Medicare ECG Law Could Be Just the First Step." *American Medical News* February 11: 1,29.

Chassin, M. R., et al. 1986. "Variations in the Use of Medical and Surgical Services by the Medicare Population." *New England Journal of Medicine* 314: 285–90.

Chassin, M. R., et al. 1987. "Does Inappropriate Use Explain Geographic Variations in the Use of Health Care Services? A Study of Three Procedures." *Journal of the American Medical Association* 258: 2533–37.

Evans, R. G., et al. 1989. "Controlling Health Expenditures—The Canadian Reality." *New England Journal of Medicine* 320: 571–77.

Ginsburg, P. B., L. B. LeRoy, and G. T. Hammons. 1990. "UpDate Medicare Physician Payment Reform." *Health Affairs* 9(1): 178–88.

Health Care Financing Administration. 1990. "Legislative Update Reports to Congress: Medicare Physician Payment." *Health Care Financing Review* 11(3): 133–42.

Holahan, J., A. Dor, and S. Zuckerman. 1990. "Understanding the Recent Growth in Medicare Physician Expenditures." *Journal of the American Medical Association* 263: 1658–61.

Holahan, J., J. Hadley, and W. Scanlon. 1979. "Paying for Physician Services under Medicare and Medicaid." *Milbank* 57(Spring): 183–211.

Iglehart, J. K. 1990. "Health Policy Report: The New Law on Medicare's Payments to Physicians." *New England Journal of Medicine* 322: 1247–52.

Kahn, K. L., J. Kosecoff, M. R. Chassin, D. H. Solomon, and R. H. Brook. 1988. "The Use and Misuse of Upper Gastrointestinal Endoscopy." *Annals of Internal Medicine* 109: 664–70.

Langwell, K. M., and L. M. Nelson. 1986. "Physician Payment Systems: A Review of History, Alternatives, and Evidence." *Medical Care Review* 43(1): 5–58.

Lee, P. R., L. B. LeRoy, P. B. Ginsberg, and G. T. Hammons. 1990. "Physician Payment Reform: An Idea Whose Time Has Come." *Medical Care Review* 47(2): 137–63.

Levy, J. M., M. J. Borowitz, S. F. Jencks, T. L. Kay, and D. K. Williams. 1990. "Impact of the Medicare Fee Schedule on Payments to Physicians." *Journal of the American Medical Association* 264: 717–22.

Office of Technology Assessment (OTA). 1986. *Payment for Physician Services: Strategies for Medicare*. OTA-H-294. Washington, DC: U.S. Government Printing Office.

Physician Payment Review Commission (PPRC). 1988. *Annual Report to Congress*. Washington, DC: PPRC.

———. 1990. *Annual Report to Congress*. Washington, DC: PPRC.

Wilensky, G. R., and L. F. Rossiter. 1986. "Alternative Units of Payment for Physician Services: An Overview of the Issues." *Medical Care Review* 43(1): 133–56.

Winslow, C. M., D. H. Solomon, M. R. Chassin, J. Kosecoff, N. J. Merrick, and R. H. Brook. 1988. "The Appropriateness of Carotid Endarterectomy." *New England Journal of Medicine* 318: 721–27.

# Chapter 2

# Payment for Medicare Physician Services

The dramatic changes in the Medicare physician payment policy enacted in 1989 speak to the perceived intractability of the steady increase in the program's costs, virtually since its inception in 1965. Interestingly, some policymakers involved in the original design of the program now say that they were well aware of the potential for unacceptably large increases in expenditures over the years, given the design of the program. But structuring a program that was locally responsive and economically attractive to physicians, and hence able to secure passage of legislation involving mainstream health care for the elderly, was the prevailing objective at the time (Cotter 1987; OTA 1986). The question of what to do if cost increases were unacceptably large was postponed for later consideration. (We will not speculate on what policymakers know but are not saying about the most recent reforms.)

The growth in expenditures that has occurred in the program has indeed been dramatic, especially in recent years. Part B spending increased an average of 8.6 percent per year, after accounting for inflation and increases in beneficiary enrollment, between 1967 and 1984 (Burney et al. 1984). From 1980 to 1989, Medicare's share of the federal budget increased from 5.2 percent to 9.1 percent (PPRC 1990). That such growth made it difficult to pay for competing social needs and to avoid tax increases became evident by the mid-1980s. In 1986, Congress appointed a high-level advisory committee, the Physician Payment Review Commission (PPRC), to study the problem and recommend solutions.

What caused this growth in costs? At least two legitimate factors, overall inflation and an increase in the size of the beneficiary population, are known to have contributed to nominal increases in Part B expenditures. But these account for only a portion of the overall increase, and that portion has diminished in recent years. Excess inflation in the medical sector has also added to Medicare expenditures, as have increases in the volume and intensity of services provided to Medicare beneficiaries. In this chapter, we examine these contributing factors in some detail to demonstrate the magnitude of their impact and the ways they have shaped the present approach to reform.

## Components of Medicare Part B Expenditure Growth

Medicare Part B spending during a given time can be expressed as a product of factors. For example, we normally think of total spending as the product of price times quantity. However, to capture the significance of volume and intensity, a somewhat different, more detailed breakdown is needed. This breakdown is given in the following equation:

Medicare       Number of beneficiaries × Services per beneficiary
Part B     =   × (Price level of Medicare services/Price level of all
spending       goods and services) × Price level of all goods and services

The first factor in total spending is simply the number of beneficiaries in a given year. This is multiplied by a measure of volume and intensity— services per beneficiary—to get the total number of services. That total is then multiplied by the relative price of medical care—that is, the price per unit of medical care relative to (divided by) the price level of all other goods and services. Finally, this quantity is multiplied again by the price level of all goods and services. Cancellation of the units of measurement shows that the final product represents the total Medicare Part B spending during the year.

This formula can also be used to break down spending growth over a period of time. For example, total Medicare Part B spending in 1990 was 21.873 times the level of spending in 1970 (Tables 2.1 and 2.2). During this ten-year period, the number of beneficiaries grew by about two-thirds over the 1970 base. The general price level, measured by the GNP deflator (an index of price levels relative to the base year of 1982), grew threefold, and medical care prices compared to all prices increased by a factor of 1.528 (Table 2.2). The last ratio indicates that medical care was about 50 percent more expensive in 1990 than in 1970, compared to other goods and services. Finally, volume and intensity change (measured as a residual, or that portion of the total change *not* attributable to prices or beneficiaries) was 2.7 times the 1970 base. The product of all four ratios is equal to 21.873, which represents the increase in total spending.

**Table 2.1**   Medicare Part B Enrollment and Spending Trends Data
from Program Inception to 1990

| Year | Enrollees (millions) | Benefits (billion $) | GNP Deflator | Medical Care Price Index |
|------|----------|----------|----------|----------|
| 1966 | 17,736 | 0.128* | 35.0 | 26.3 |
| 1967 | 17,893 | 1.197 | 35.9 | 28.2 |
| 1968 | 18,805 | 1.518 | 37.7 | 29.9 |
| 1969 | 19,195 | 1.865 | 39.8 | 31.9 |
| 1970 | 19,584 | 1.975 | 42.0 | 34.0 |
| 1971 | 19,975 | 2.117 | 44.4 | 36.1 |
| 1972 | 20,351 | 2.325 | 46.5 | 37.3 |
| 1973 | 22,491 | 2.526 | 49.5 | 38.8 |
| 1974 | 23,167 | 3.318 | 54.0 | 42.4 |
| 1975 | 23,905 | 4.273 | 59.3 | 47.5 |
| 1976 | 24,614 | 5.080 | 63.1 | 52.0 |
| 1977 | 25,364 | 6.038 | 67.3 | 57.0 |
| 1978 | 26,074 | 7.252 | 72.2 | 61.8 |
| 1979 | 26,757 | 8.708 | 78.6 | 67.5 |
| 1980 | 27,400 | 10.635 | 85.7 | 74.9 |
| 1981 | 27,941 | 13.113 | 94.0 | 82.9 |
| 1982 | 28,412 | 15.455 | 100.0 | 92.5 |
| 1983 | 28,974 | 18.106 | 103.9 | 100.6 |
| 1984 | 29,415 | 19.661 | 107.9 | 106.8 |
| 1985 | 29,989 | 22.947 | 110.9 | 113.5 |
| 1986 | 30,590 | 26.239 | 113.8 | 122.0 |
| 1987 | 31,170 | 30.820 | 117.4 | 130.1 |
| 1988 | 31,600 | 33.970 | 121.3 | 138.6 |
| 1989 | 32,100† | 37.200 | 126.3 | 149.3 |
| 1990 | 32,800† | 43.200 | 131.5 | 162.8 |

*Sources:* Enrollment (as of July 1) through 1982 from *Health Care Financing Program Statistics, Medicare and Medicaid Data Book* (Washington, DC: HCFA, 1986), Table 2.1; 1983–88 from *Social Security Bulletin, Annual Statistical Supplement* (Washington, DC: U.S. GPO, 1989), Table 7.B1 and p. 3; 1989–90 from *1990 HCFA Statistics* (Washington, DC: HCFA, 1990), Tables 1 and 2.

Benefit outlays through 1988 from *Social Security Bulletin, Annual Statistical Supplement* (Washington, DC: U.S. GPO, 1989), Table 7.A2; 1989–90 from *1990 HCFA Statistics* (Washington, DC: HCFA, 1990), Table 27.

GNP deflator and medical care price index from *Economic Report of the President, 1991* (Washington, DC: U.S. GPO, 1991), Tables B-3 and B-58.

*1966 benefits are for July–December only.
†1989–1990 enrollment data are estimated.

**Table 2.2**  Factors That Contribute to Medicare Part B Spending and Spending Levels at End of Period Relative to Beginning of Period, 1970 to 1990

| Factors | 1970–1990 | 1970–1975 | 1975–1980 | 1980–1985 | 1985–1990 |
|---|---|---|---|---|---|
| Part B spending | 21.873 | 2.164 | 2.489 | 2.158 | 1.883 |
| Enrollment | 1.675 | 1.221 | 1.146 | 1.094 | 1.094 |
| General inflation | 3.131 | 1.412 | 1.445 | 1.294 | 1.186 |
| Medical care inflation | 1.528 | 0.989 | 1.091 | 1.170 | 1.210 |
| Volume and intensity | 2.724 | 1.266 | 1.378 | 1.301 | 1.200 |

We can also calculate the percentage contribution made by each factor to the rise in total spending (Table 2.3). Over the 1970–1990 period, general inflation made the largest contribution to Medicare Part B spending growth, accounting for 37.0 percent. This was followed by volume and intensity, which accounted for 32.5 percent of spending growth. Enrollment growth was a distant third factor, accounting for only 16.7 percent of total spending growth. Finally, medical care inflation in excess of general inflation was the least important factor, contributing 13.7 percent to total spending growth.

Some interesting trends emerge when we examine the five-year periods indicated in Table 2.3. First, enrollment growth was a more important factor in the early years (1970–1975) of the Medicare program, when it accounted for about one-fourth of spending growth. Since then, its contribution has been smaller and shows no apparent trend. Second, the contribution of volume and intensity was highest in the middle two periods and lowest in the last five-year period. Third, general inflation plays a decreasingly important role over time, with a contribution that declines

**Table 2.3**  Percentage Contribution of Various Factors to Rising Medicare Part B Spending, 1970 to 1990

| Factors | 1970–1990 (%) | 1970–1975 (%) | 1975–1980 (%) | 1980–1985 (%) | 1985–1990 (%) |
|---|---|---|---|---|---|
| Enrollment | 16.7 | 25.9 | 14.9 | 11.7 | 14.2 |
| General inflation | 37.0 | 44.7 | 40.4 | 33.6 | 27.0 |
| Medical care inflation | 13.7 | −1.4 | 9.5 | 20.4 | 30.2 |
| Volume and intensity | 32.5 | 30.6 | 35.2 | 34.2 | 28.8 |

*Note:* Columns may not total 100.0% due to rounding.

in each five-year period from 1970 to 1990. Offsetting the decline in the importance of general inflation is an increasing role for medical care inflation, which accounted for 30.2 percent of the increase in spending over the last five-year period.

Because medical care policymakers can do nothing to control enrollment or general inflation, it appears that only about 60 percent of Medicare Part B spending is, in principle, controllable. In the 1985–1990 period, the controllable increase was divided almost equally between volume and intensity growth and medical care price inflation that exceeds general inflation. This distribution represents a substantial change from the earlier periods in which medical price inflation was much less important and volume and intensity growth dominated.

The sections that follow focus on what is known about the factors that influence the relative magnitude of each of the components of Part B expenditure growth except general inflation. The impacts of both the customary, prevailing, and reasonable (CPR) method of payment and the growing number of beneficiaries on Medicare expenditure increases are discussed briefly. Issues surrounding the increase in volume and intensity of services suggested by the growth in the residual are also addressed. Certain problems with the residual as a measure of volume and intensity are noted, and a number of factors that could have fueled increases in the number and sophistication of services to Medicare patients are considered. These factors include certain Medicare policies themselves, a growing demand for health care by the elderly, and increasingly sophisticated technology.

**Excess inflation in Medicare: Is CPR payment to blame?**

Customary, prevailing, and reasonable reimbursement is based on physician charges for individual services provided. The CPR approach is specific to Medicare and is similar to the usual, customary, and reasonable (UCR) payment approach used in many private insurance plans. Under the guidelines of CPR payment, when a physician submits a charge for a service provided to a Medicare beneficiary, the *reasonable* charge (i.e., what is actually paid) is the lowest of the customary charge, the prevailing charge, and the physician's actual charge for the service. The *customary* charge is the physician's median charge for the same service in the previous year. The *prevailing* charge is a predetermined percentile of the customary charges for the service by all physicians in a geographic area (OTA 1986; Cotter 1987).

Because of the way the "pure" CPR system works, submission of a high fee in the current year, although it does not result in a higher immediate payment, will increase both customary and prevailing charges, setting the stage for higher reasonable (actual) payments in the next year. The CPR reimbursement method thus encourages physicians to increase their fees continually. The primary constraint under Medicare's original CPR scheme was, paradoxically, the requirement that doctors match higher fees to Medicare patients with higher fees to their non-Medicare patients. The requirement was established with the hope that the latter would be unwilling to pay the higher price.

The rapid expenditure growth experienced during the early years of the Medicare program was thought to be at least partly attributable to this method of payment, so various controls were put on fee increases in an attempt to contain aggregate costs. In 1971 and 1972, the economywide price controls of the Nixon administration were left on physician charges for 15 months after they were lifted elsewhere (Cotter 1987). The Medicare economic index was introduced in 1975 to restrain yearly increases in prevailing fees to a level in keeping with economywide inflation and the actual practice costs that physicians faced. The MEI measures increases in general earnings levels and in physician practice costs; thus, it is a measure of yearly increases in input prices (OTA 1986). With the use of the MEI, the prevailing charge used to determine payment for a specific service is the lesser of either the unadjusted prevailing charge or the product of the 1973 prevailing charge for the service in question multiplied by the value of the current MEI (OTA 1986). For the majority of physicians who are constrained by the MEI, the inflationary potential of the "customary" part of the CPR payment was thus eliminated. The other major control on Medicare physician fees was the freeze of 1984–1986, which was mandated by the Deficit Reduction Act of 1984. (The fee freeze is discussed in detail later in this chapter.)

### Increases in beneficiary enrollment

The aging of the American population has certainly contributed to growth in Medicare expenditures over the years. One would anticipate this demographic change to affect program costs in two ways: First, the increasing number of persons over the age of 65 would be expected to result in an increase in enrollment in Part B. Second, the increasing number of old elderly might lead to a greater demand for more services.

Relative to other factors, however, these specific demographic changes appear to have become less important in recent years. Increasing enrollment was a major contributor to increases in spending in the early years of the program but has become less important over time. In addition, one recent study suggests that the old elderly actually appear to use fewer services than the young elderly (Holahan, Dor, and Zuckerman 1990). Thus, these demographic influences in and of themselves seem to be relatively minor factors in overall Part B expenditure growth. As the baby boom generation retires, however, demographic changes will eventually dominate Part B spending growth.

The CPR method of payment and the growing number of Medicare beneficiaries have contributed to the spending increases witnessed in Part B over the years. However, overall costs continued to rise in the face of controls on fee levels, in excess even of what was expected given the growing number of beneficiaries. Thus, it is apparent that the number and complexity of services provided *per beneficiary* increased as well. There were many factors working throughout the 1960s, 1970s, and 1980s that could have contributed to this phenomenon.

### Residual Part B growth: Volume and intensity changes

It is generally agreed that the portion of Part B expenditure growth not attributable to inflation or enrollment is the result of increases in either the volume or the mix (that is, the intensity) of physician services. Many factors could contribute to growing volume and intensity of care. Before examining these, however, it is important to identify some of the weaknesses of this residual as a measure of volume and intensity, and to understand what it really tells us.

Volume and intensity growth is not measured directly; it is measured indirectly as a residual. Specifically, it is the portion of the yearly increase in Part B expenditures that cannot be explained by economywide inflation, excess inflation in medical prices (as measured by the consumer price index for the medical sector, or CPI-Med, which is a measure of output prices), and growth in beneficiary enrollment. Because it is an indirect measure, it tells little about whether services have truly increased in number, whether they have become more complex, or whether they have simply been unbundled and charged for separately instead of being provided as a package (Falk and Langwell 1988). Because the residual depends on measures of fee growth, it is heavily influenced by the CPI-Med, which measures a set of charges for all health care services, not just those in Medicare. And significant differences may exist.[1] Further, the residual fails to take into account increases in the number of Medicare enrollees who actually use services; if more are using services, overall growth may be appropriate and may not represent an increase in the volume or intensity of services per user (Falk and Langwell 1988). Finally, year-to-year changes in the residual have been somewhat erratic. Because there is no logical reason to expect yearly increases in the volume or intensity of services to fluctuate substantially, errors in measurement of changes in fee levels may be causing the apparent residual to gyrate. Some doubt is therefore cast on the residual's validity as a short-run measure of volume and intensity changes (Falk and Langwell 1988).

The factors that could contribute to increases in the number and complexity of services that physicians provide to Medicare beneficiaries include certain Medicare policies themselves, a growing demand for health care by the elderly, and a desire by both patients and physicians for increasingly sophisticated technology. An overview of each of these and of the actual evidence of their impact on the volume and intensity of care follows. Much of this evidence comes from two major studies conducted to assess the causes and components of Medicare spending growth during the mid-1980s—one by Mitchell, Wedig, and Cromwell (1989), and another by Holahan, Dor, and Zuckerman (1990). Because both studies used multivariate techniques, the effects of a range of factors on Part B costs were estimated. The results shed some light on the reasons behind the rapid growth in Medicare expenditures on physician services.

### Medicare policies of the 1980s

The political attractiveness of protecting the elderly from the health care cost increases of the 1980s resulted in three major policy changes during the decade, prior to the enactment in 1989 of the Medicare fee schedule with volume performance standards. The first was the implementation of the prospective payment system (PPS) within the Medicare program's hospital insurance program (Medicare Part A), which was phased in beginning in October 1983. This policy changed the reimbursement system for hospital care from a cost-based method to a system based on a fixed price per diagnosis (regardless of actual costs), analogous to a fee schedule.

The Deficit Reduction Act (DEFRA) of 1984 mandated the other two new policies. The first of these was the Medicare Participating Physician and Supplier Program, which rewarded physicians for agreeing to participate by accepting assignment (i.e., Medicare payment in full) for their Medicare patients. DEFRA also mandated a freeze on physicians' fees, which began in June 1984 and continued for participating physicians through April 1986 and for nonparticipating physicians through December 1986 (Cotter 1987).

*The prospective payment system.*    The incentives offered and changes wrought by the prospective payment system are, by now, reasonably well documented. The PPS pays a predetermined price, based on diagnosis, for each Medicare-covered hospitalization. When the actual costs of caring for any beneficiary during a given hospitalization exceed this predetermined price, the hospital is financially responsible for the excess amount. If actual costs are less than the Medicare payment, the hospital retains the difference. Intended to stimulate efficiency by reducing the level of services and shortening lengths of stay, PPS provides hospitals with incentives to minimize costs per admission. At least two strategies can be used to accomplish this. The first strategy is to avoid hospitalization of money-losing cases, perhaps by providing care to the severely ill costly patient on an outpatient basis. With the exception (since 1989) of outpatient surgery, outpatient care is still reimbursed on a cost basis. The second strategy is to minimize the number of hospital days and services. The first strategy is generally implausible because the acutely sick high-cost patients within a diagnosis-related group (DRG) category could not easily be treated in an outpatient setting. One way of using the second strategy however, is to provide as many services as possible on an outpatient basis prior or subsequent to hospitalization. Diagnostic testing and rehabilitation, for example, can often be provided on an outpatient basis rather than as part of a hospitalization. Some analysts suggest that the trend toward providing care in office settings reflects this strategy. An alternative theory suggests that the shift to office settings may be the response of physicians frustrated by hospital limits on resources per stay (Pauly and Kissick 1988).

Implementation of PPS appears to have been associated with decreased admission rates and lengths of stay, both of which have contributed to moderation in Part A expenditures (Russell 1989; Feder, Hadley, and Zuckerman 1987; Holahan, Dor, and Zuckerman 1990; PPRC 1990). In a review of changes in the patterns of care associated with PPS, Russell (1989) reports a number of facts that are consistent with a "PPS effect." In the first year of prospective hospital payment (1983–1984), Medicare admissions decreased by just over 1 percent, from approximately 10.4 million to 10.3 million. Admissions per beneficiary continued to decline through 1986. Over the next two years admissions rose modestly, but to a level still well below that of 1983. Lengths of hospital stays for Medicare beneficiaries decreased from 9.7 days to 8.6 days in the first year of PPS and have changed little since then. According to Russell, much of the change in admissions can be traced to shifts in surgery from inpatient to outpatient settings. The shift to outpatient surgery for cataract surgery alone accounted for slightly over half of the total decline in admissions between 1984 and 1985. Sloan, Morrisey, and Valvona (1988a) attributed the drop in admissions to scrutiny by PPS-related professional review organizations, rather than to financial incentives per se.

Russell also provides evidence that services previously provided in the hospital have been shifted to other settings as a result of PPS. She and others have cited data showing that preoperative lengths of stay for Medicare patients dropped from 3.1 days in 1983 to 2.7 days in 1984 and remained at the lower level in 1985 (Russell 1989; DesHarnais et al. 1987). It has also been suggested that the rate of growth in inpatient testing dropped even more sharply than admissions (Sloan, Morrisey, and Valvona 1988b; Russell 1989). The number of inpatients receiving bone scans, for example, which had been growing by 6 percent per year prior to PPS, decreased 15 percent per year in the first two years of PPS. Several other tests were shown to have followed similar patterns.

But what is the effect of PPS on Part B costs? As noted earlier, some increases in Part B expenditures may have resulted from the PPS-induced shifting of services such as testing and rehabilitation to outpatient settings, and from the substitution of physician services for hospital services (Mitchell, Wedig, and Cromwell 1989; Holahan, Dor, and Zuckerman 1990). It is therefore important to assess the extent to which PPS contributed to rising Part B costs in the 1980s.

Research findings on the effects of PPS on Part B expenditures and volume are not clear-cut. Recall that Part B has always paid for physician services, whether delivered in the hospital or elsewhere, as well as for certain other services provided in nonhospital settings. Because there is no conclusive reason why PPS should increase the overall demand for physician services (in fact, it could even decrease the opportunity to provide physician services because of shortened lengths of stay and fewer admissions), the shift in care away from the hospital would be expected to increase Part B costs only to the extent that these other services (e.g., laboratory studies and radiographs) are now provided outside of the hospital and charged to Part B, whereas previously they had been provided as part of hospitalization and charged to Part A.

There is no question but that the implementation of PPS coincided with a shift in services from hospitals to nonhospital settings such as outpatient departments of hospitals, physicians' offices, and independent laboratories. Charges for physician services provided in the hospital fell from 61 percent of Part B charges in 1982 to 47 percent in 1986, whereas those for physician services provided in hospital outpatient departments increased from about 5 percent to nearly 16 percent over the same period. Physician services provided in office-based and other nonhospital settings increased as well, but to a lesser extent (Russell 1989). However, because Part B pays for physician services regardless of where they are provided, the question remains as to whether PPS caused other nonhospital services to increase significantly enough to contribute to the overall growth in Part B expenditures. Physician services account for approximately 73 percent of all Part B costs so a fairly dramatic increase in the remaining 27 percent of services would be needed to produce any significant growth in Part B expenditures overall (PPRC 1990; Russell 1989.)

In their study using data from 1983 and 1985 on services and expenditures for a 5 percent sample of Medicare beneficiaries, Holahan, Dor, and Zuckerman (1990) noted that, because of the decrease in hospital admissions and lengths of stay, physician services appeared to decrease approximately 2.3 percent between the two years. At the same time, the shifting of other services to Part B caused an increase in expenditures of about 4.2 percent. They concluded that PPS was statistically insignificant as a determinant of the increase in Part B volume and intensity from 1983 to 1985. Their assessment, then, was that the prospective payment system appeared to have been a fairly minor contributor to the residual growth in Part B costs.

Mitchell, Wedig, and Cromwell (1989) also considered the impact of PPS on Part B costs, but their results suggest a somewhat greater effect. Using Part B data from four representative Medicare carrier regions (Alabama, Connecticut, Washington, and Wisconsin) over the four years from 1983 through 1986, they found that there may have been a lagged effect of PPS. That is, in the short run, PPS may have caused a decrease in Part B expenditures, but over the longer term the quantity of Part B services increased. The authors speculated that such an effect could be caused not only by the substitution of physician care for hospital care but also by the growth in outpatient technologies and facilities as a result of continued reimbursement on a cost basis. These effects plausibly might have been delayed, because it takes time to establish new referral patterns, develop and disseminate technologies, and build new facilities. Mitchell, Wedig, and Cromwell estimated that PPS was responsible for as much as one-half of the increase in the quantity of Part B services provided over the study period.

Taken together, these results hint that physician and nonphysician services were shifted from the hospital to various nonhospital settings following the implementation of PPS. The effects of PPS on the actual volume of physician services and on overall Part B costs, however, remain unclear. Focusing on a shorter time period, the analysis by Holahan, Dor, and Zuckerman revealed a decrease in physician services and a negligible overall increase in Part B costs (owing to the shift in other services to outpatient settings) subsequent to the initiation of PPS. However, the results of Mitchell, Wedig, and Cromwell's longer-term study suggest that after a lag period, overall Part B services and costs may have increased in response to PPS. Mitchell's team found this effect to be fairly strong, with PPS responsible for about 50 percent of the volume growth over the period, so Part B volume increases caused by PPS could have contributed to the overall expenditure increases of the mid-1980s.

*The physician fee freeze of 1984–1986.* Having addressed Medicare's growing hospital costs by implementing the prospective payment system (and thereby potentially stimulating physician services), Congress chose to focus on the expanding Part B expenditures by mandating the DEFRA physician fee freeze of 1984. This freeze on customary and prevailing charges eliminated two anticipated fee updates for participating physicians and three for nonparticipating doctors. During the period of this fee freeze (1984–1986), however, Part B expenditures continued to increase, prompting speculation that physicians had somehow increased the number or complexity of services provided so as to maintain income (Mitchell, Wedig, and Cromwell 1989).

The DEFRA fee freeze presents some particularly intriguing questions regarding cause and effect. If fees decrease in real terms (as they did during the freeze, when held constant in the face of inflation), will physicians provide fewer services because they receive a lower price? Will they act as "income targeters" and simply provide more services to achieve the same income as before? Or will beneficiary demand increase because of the lower real out-of-pocket costs and higher pension payments to beneficiaries?

Other Medicare policy changes implemented at about the same time (such as the PPS, the participating provider program, and direct billing for laboratory services) complicate assessment of the causal impact of the fee freeze itself, making empirical evidence on what actually happened to volume and intensity as a result of the freeze ambiguous.

To explore the determinants of rising overall expenditures in the face of the fee freeze, Mitchell, Wedig, and Cromwell, using the same four-state data set described above, first constructed a price index using a "market basket" of five common services for each physician specialty. Each service was then aggregated across specialties, and nominal expenditures were adjusted for inflation to arrive at *real* expenditures per beneficiary—a measure of volume and intensity growth. Real expenditures per beneficiary, measured in this way, rose approximately 11 percent during the fee freeze. The fee freeze was not found to be the primary cause of this increase in volume, however. Only about one-fifth of the total increase in volume and intensity was attributed to the freeze, with as much as one-half of the increase attributed to implementation of the prospective payment system (Mitchell, Wedig, and Cromwell 1988).

Holahan, Dor, and Zuckerman (1990) also examined the effect of the fee freeze on volume. They estimated that during their study period (1983 to 1985) nominal expenditures per enrollee increased by almost

15 percent, with only about 4 percentage points of this increase attributable to price increases, leaving nearly 11 percentage points resulting from volume and intensity growth. Holahan, Dor, and Zuckerman, like Mitchell, Wedig, and Cromwell, estimated that the freeze itself was not a major influence on volume since it appeared to have caused less than 10 percent of the growth in volume and intensity that occurred between 1983 and 1985. Other factors were found to be more important to Part B volume growth; these include physician participation in the Medicare program (discussed in more detail below), increasing incomes of the elderly, and new technologies (although the researchers noted that the last two factors may be related in the sense that expensive new technologies may disseminate more rapidly in higher-income markets). They also concluded that physicians did not increase service volumes in response to the freeze and that the freeze did, in fact, realize its intended goal. Part B volume and expenditures would have been higher had it not been for the freeze.

Based on these studies, it appears that the DEFRA fee freeze of 1984 was not a significant factor in the volume and intensity growth of this period. The studies do not provide conclusive evidence of income-targeting behavior among physicians.

*The Participating Physician and Supplier Program.* The final policy change of the 1980s occurred during the latter stages of the fee freeze with the implementation of the Medicare Participating Physician and Supplier Program. Intended to further protect beneficiaries from the increasing costs of care, this program's effect was to decrease the elderly's out-of-pocket costs. Because it lowered the price of care in this way, it was also suspected of stimulating the demand for services and of fueling an increase in volume and intensity of care during this time.

How do "participation" and "assignment" work? In the early years of Medicare, physicians were given the option of accepting assignment, that is, accepting Medicare's payment as payment in full, on a per service basis. If assignment was accepted, the physician was prohibited from billing the patient for any charge in excess of that amount. Initially, approximately 60 percent of all Medicare claims were paid in this way (Lee et al. 1990). By 1978, however, this rate had fallen to about 51 percent, as physicians responded to price controls imposed by the Nixon administration in the early 1970s and to limits (resulting from the use of the Medicare economic index) on annual fee updates (Mitchell and Cromwell 1982; Lee et al. 1990; Ferry et al. 1980; McMenamin 1987).

To increase these assignment rates, Congress enacted the Medicare Participating Physician and Supplier Program in 1984 (OTA 1986; Cotter 1987). Participation in the program, which now required that a physician sign an agreement to accept assignment on all of his or her Medicare patients, was encouraged by allowing annual updates in the charges of participating physicians and denying them to nonparticipating physicians.

These financial incentives for participation appear to have been effective. During the first quarter of the participating provider program, assignment rates increased by nearly 5 percent (McMenamin 1987). As of 1988, approximately 81 percent of services were provided on assignment (Lee et al. 1990). It is important to note, however, that independent laboratories had been required to accept assignment in 1984, as had physician office labs in 1987; so not all of the increase in assignment rates was for physician services (PPRC 1988).

What were the program's consequences for Part B volume and intensity? Based on economic theory, one would predict that decreasing the out-of-pocket expenses of beneficiaries would increase the quantity of services demanded. Holahan et al. (1990) estimated that the decrease in cost sharing was the most important factor in volume growth during the fee freeze of the 1980s, and that it was responsible for approximately one-fourth of the growth in volume and intensity between 1983 and 1985. Medicare policies themselves appear, therefore, to have contributed to the Part B volume and expenditure increases of the 1980s. The prospective payment system seems to have shifted services to the outpatient setting and perhaps stimulated outpatient technologies, resulting in increased Part B costs. By decreasing out-of-pocket expenses for Medicare beneficiaries, the physician participation program helped stimulate demand for covered services. The extent to which the demand for care has influenced Part B costs is considered in the following section.

### Growing demand for health care

Since well before the advent of Medicare, Americans have increasingly demanded comprehensive, sophisticated health care. Advances in technology, and the growth of widespread insurance coverage to pay for that technology, have caused patients and physicians to become accustomed to more rather than less care and services. The elderly prove to be no exception to this general rule, and as a group, they have become increasingly able to afford extensive (and expensive) health care. Medicare, of course, pays for the majority of their health care costs, but for some expensive illnesses the portion left for the beneficiary to pay can be burdensome. The financial support of Social Security benefits, as well as growing wealth from other sources, have enabled most of the elderly to purchase Medigap insurance policies to cover much of the expense not paid by Medicare. Nearly 70 percent of beneficiaries have these policies; another 13 percent have similar coverage through Medicaid (HCFA 1985).

By decreasing the out-of-pocket costs to the patient and dissociating the cost of care from the actual services received, such extensive insurance coverage is thought to stimulate the demand for care.

Is there evidence to support this assumption? Holahan, Dor, and Zuckerman (1990) found that the incomes of the elderly had grown by more than 13 percent per capita during the years of their study (1983 to 1985), and that this increase accounted for another one-fourth of the growth in the volume and intensity of services delivered to Medicare benficiaries. Although this explanation has not been tested for the entire period of Medicare Part B expenditure growth, it does seem plausible that the erosion of the Part B cost sharing through the expanded Medigap coverage made possible by higher incomes is a likely cause of expenditure growth.

### Sophisticated, expensive technology

Given the willingness and ability of many Medicare patients to consume health care resources and the physician's desire to be maximally effective, doctors have tended over the years to provide services that *might* be useful in a given clinical situation, regardless of the degree to which they are likely or proven to be successful. The growing sophistication of health care technology has made improved technology an increasingly expensive proposition. Consequently, the advances in technology that have occurred in the past decade have come to be seen as a key factor in the growing intensity of care. Research on the expenditure increases of the 1980s has made clearer the extent to which Medicare spending is driven by the use of technology and the technological changes in care.

In both studies of the Part B expenditure increases that occurred in the mid-1980s, the role of technology in volume and intensity increases was found to be significant. As noted earlier, Mitchell, Wedig, and Cromwell (1989) found that during the freeze on fees, spending for physician services increased by 26 percent. Some of this increase was caused by fee updates that had occurred prior to the freeze and by fee updates made for participating physicians while the freeze was extended for nonparticipating doctors. Even after accounting for these factors, however, there remained a 22 percent increase in spending that seemed to be caused by growth in the number and kind of physician services provided.

Mitchell, Wedig, and Cromwell (1989) found that most of the increase in spending represented payment for a few surgeries and procedures. The number of cataract surgeries performed, for example, increased by 50 percent, largely because of the development of an implantable intraocular lens that significantly improved the outcomes of cataract surgery. This technology also changed the surgery into a more sophisticated procedure; whereas earlier treatment consisted of simple extraction of the affected lens, physicians could now essentially restore vision by implanting an artificial lens. Similarly, because diffusion of improved fiberoptic endoscopes enabled better visualization of the colon and upper gastrointestinal tract, procedures involving these technologies became more commonly used as diagnostic tools. Utilization rates for colonoscopies more than doubled between 1983 and 1986; those for sigmoidoscopies tripled. Increases in the use of diagnostic cardiac services, coronary artery bypass graft surgery, total knee replacements, inguinal hernia repairs, and total hip replacements followed similar, if somewhat less dramatic, patterns.

The study by Holahan, Dor, and Zuckerman (1990) seemed to corroborate these findings. The authors described marked increases in payments to the physician specialties in which several of these procedures are used: ophthalmology, radiology, and orthopedic surgery. They concluded that much of the growth in volume and intensity of care during 1983 and 1985 was caused by changes in technology. It would appear, therefore, that the development and spread of new technologies is a major factor that has driven Part B costs. This is, perhaps, to be expected, considering the relatively high payments for these technical procedures under CPR reimbursement.

## Summary

The data cited here strongly suggest that the number and mix of services provided to Medicare beneficiaries did increase during the 1980s. Although there was no evidence of growth in the volume of services of no benefit, there was growth in certain effective procedural services made possible by beneficial new technologies for which payment was relatively generous. It is no surprise, then, that Congress aimed the present reforms at both redistribution of prices and overall restraint of services. It is perhaps equally unsurprising that, given the strong demand for effective sophisticated care, Congress has not indicated how it wishes physicians to ration costly but beneficial new technologies in the future.

The evidence on factors that drive physician and outpatient costs must, of course, be considered preliminary. More studies of the actual nature of the residual and its behavior over time are needed to guide future policies aimed at restraining it. Some of these studies must be evaluations of the effect of the present reforms on costs and services in general and on the residual in particular. Consideration of the behavioral and economic theories presented in this book, and of the effects of other controls on volume and intensity, should be useful to these future research and policy efforts.

# Note

1. This issue is addressed by some, notably the Physician Payment Review Commission, by using Medicare allowed charges, rather than the CPI-Med, as a measure of price increases (PPRC 1990).

# References

Burney, I., P. Hickman, J. Paradise, and G. Schieber. 1984. "Medicare Physician Payment, Participation, and Reform." *Health Affairs* 3(4): 5–24.

Cotter, P. S. 1987. *Physician Service Coverage under Medicare: History, Performance, and Evaluation.* Chicago: American Medical Association, Center for Health Policy Research.

DesHarnais, S., E. Kobrinski, J. Chesney, M. Long, R. Ament, and S. Fleming. 1987. "The Early Effects of the Prospective Payment System on Inpatient Utilization and the Quality of Care." *Inquiry* 24: 7–16.

Falk, G., and K. Langwell. 1988. *Growth in the Volume of Medicare Physician Services: A Framework for Analysis.* Washington, DC: Congressional Research Service, Library of Congress.

Feder, J., J. Hadley, and S. Zuckerman. 1987. "How Did Medicare's Prospective Payment System Affect Hospitals?" *New England Journal of Medicine* 317: 867–73.

Ferry, T. P., M. Gornick, M. Newton, and C. Hackerman. 1980. "Physicians' Charges under Medicare: Assignment Rates and Beneficiary Liability." *Health Care Financing Review* 1(3): 49–73.

Health Care Financing Administration (HCFA). Office of Research and Demonstration. 1985. "Supplemental Health Insurance Coverage among Aged Medicare Beneficiaries." In *National Medical Care Utilization and Expenditure Survey.* Series B, Descriptive Report No. 5. DHHS Publication No. 85-20205. Washington, DC: National Center for Health Services Research.

Holahan, J., A. Dor, and S. Zuckerman. 1990. "Understanding the Recent Growth in Medicare Physician Expenditures." *Journal of the American Medical Association* 263: 1658–61.

Lee, P. R., L. B. LeRoy, P. B. Ginsberg, and G. T. Hammons. 1990. "Physician Payment Reform: An Idea Whose Time Has Come." *Medical Care Review* 47(2): 137–63.

McMenamin, P. 1987. "Medicare Part B: Rising Assignment Rates, Rising Costs. Symposium Report." *Inquiry* 24: 344–59.

Mitchell, J. B., and J. Cromwell. 1982. "Physician Behavior under the Medicare Assignment Option." *Journal of Health Economics* 1: 245–64.

Mitchell, J. B., G. Wedig, and J. Cromwell. 1988. *Impact of the Medicare Fee Freeze on Physician Expenditures and Volumes.* HCFA Grant #15-C-98387/1. Washington, DC: Health Care Financing Administration.

———. 1989. "The Medicare Physician Fee Freeze: What Really Happened?" *Health Affairs* 8(1): 21–33.

Office of Technology Assessment (OTA). 1986. *Payment for Physician Services Strategies for Medicare.* OTA-H-294. Washington, DC: U.S. Government Printing Office.

Pauly, M. V., and W. L. Kissick, eds. 1988. *Lessons from the First Twenty Years of Medicare: Research Implications for Public and Private Sector Policy.* Philadelphia: University of Pennsylvania Press.

Physician Payment Review Commission (PPRC). 1988. *Annual Report to Congress.* Washington, DC: PPRC.

———. 1990. *Annual Report to Congress.* Washington, DC: PPRC.

Russell, L. B. 1989. *Medicare's New Hospital Payment System: Is It Working?* Washington, DC: The Brookings Institution.

Sloan, F. A., M. A. Morrisey, and J. Valvona. 1988a. "Hospital Care for the 'Self-Pay' Patient." *Journal of Health Politics, Policy and Law* 13: 83–102.

———. 1988b. "Medicare Prospective Payment and the Use of Medical Technologies in Hospitals." *Medical Care* 26: 837–53.

Chapter 3

# Models of Physician Behavior

Physicians are paid for their services as an incentive for them to furnish the particular services that patients need. Yet there are reasons to doubt that the volume of services Medicare patients receive is ideal. Some services might be provided even though they are known to cause more harm than good or to do no good at all. Other services might have small benefits but high costs. To influence volume, two broad policy options are possible. Prices or payment mechanisms could be adjusted so that they would, at some point and in some fashion, affect volume. Nonprice controls could be imposed that would supercede the decisions that doctors and patients might make regarding the provision of care. But neither Medicare nor any other insurer can review and dictate the process of care in every patient-physician encounter. To forecast the effects of various price and nonprice volume-affecting schemes, therefore, some assumptions must be made about how doctors and patients behave.

An essential element in making assumptions about physician be-havior with some degree of confidence is having some idea of what physicians are trying to do. What objectives are they trying to pursue when they produce and sell services to patients? This chapter provides three models or concepts of physician behavior that can help in pre-dicting the broader effects of various volume and price controls: the profit maximization model, the sophisticated target-income model, and the patient agency model.

## Profit Maximization Model

The simplest description for this model of physician behavior is that doctors are like other small business owners: they try to maximize profits, within the limits of whatever work effort they undertake. This does not preclude ethical behavior or concern for patients, especially if ethical behavior will encourage demand. It does imply, however, at least as a simplification, that decisions are made largely according to their effect on the bottom line over the long term. Notwithstanding doubts that physicians actually behave exactly this way, the model does provide a benchmark, a pure case of what someone with solely financial objectives might do, and therefore can serve as a stylized predictor of what effect financial incentives will have on a physician's practice.

A key behavior in this type of model is what is called "demand inducement," whereby physicians encourage patients to demand larger quantities of services at a given price (three follow-up chest x-rays instead of two, for instance). To discuss outcomes using a model in which physicians are only interested in profits and in which demand inducement is possible, we obviously need to characterize the reaction patients might have to inducement. After all, if there is no negative reaction from patients, the amount of demand inducement possible for a profitable service would be infinite. We assume that the services for which doctors are paid have independent demands, and that there is a maximum amount of service that patients can accept. That is, we imagine that different services are used to treat different illnesses (even though some are provided by the same doctor), and that there is a limit to the amount of any service a patient would accept for a particular type of illness.

## Profit maximization and the effect of price on volume

Profit is the difference between revenue and cost. For an owner-managed firm, such as a medical practice, "cost" includes not only explicit cash payments made to others for inputs but also the money value of the owner's time spent working in the business. The simplest strategy for determining the cost of owner-provided time is to price it at some valuation per hour, in much the fashion that the Urban Institute researchers did in constructing a geographic economic index of physician practice costs (Zuckerman, Welch, and Pope 1988).

When nominal output prices are frozen and real output prices fall in an inflationary environment, how would a profit-maximizing practice respond? The answer is straightforward: with no objectives other than profit, the practice would decide to sell less output (i.e., in this case, to reduce the volume of services provided and save the cost of the physician's time or other input costs). Before the price cut, the physician(s) would have been willing to sell output up to the point at which the last unit's cost had just been covered by the price received from Medicare. But were Medicare to cut its payment price, this last unit would become a money loser, and it (and some other units in the same situation) would therefore not be sold.

A critical assumption behind this commonsense conclusion is that the price cut has to force the price for some services below cost. If the initial price were substantially above cost, the quantity was constrained by demand, and the cut just pushed the price closer to cost (but not below), then the commonsense conclusion would not follow. A practice interested only in profit would continue to provide a service even if it became less profitable, so long as some money was still to be made. The real question then is how many services would shift from "gainers" to "losers" as a result of a particular price reduction. Some physicians would probably always provide some of these services just at the margin and presumably would be unwilling to continue treating Medicare patients in the same way if the price fell. The empirical issue is how wide this margin is. What is unequivocal is that price cuts to a profit-motivated supplier would either reduce volume or, in the extreme, have almost no effect on volume. According to this scenario, price cuts alone would certainly not lead to an increase in the volume of services provided.

## Adding inducement

One might suppose that the profit-seeking physician would try to recoup some of the lost total profit from services with a positive profit, even if that profit had been reduced by a price cut. The physician would only need to create further demand for the profitable service to increase the profit. Surprisingly, this is not a logical conclusion. Were the physician only interested in profit, were he or she always trying to make the profit as large as it could be, and were it possible to create demand, then according to the profit maximization theory, all profitable demand would have been created even prior to the price change. There would be no profitable niches left to be tapped. Put slightly differently, maximizing profit by creating demand implies exploitation of all profitable opportunities before the real price is cut. Because the price cut does not create any *new* opportunities for profit, nothing more is left to be exploited. In this scenario, all the gains from Medicare and the consumer have been wrung out of the system before the price cut.

This counterintuitive conclusion is sufficient to suggest that another explanation needs to be developed in which doctors have other, more noble or complex objectives than profit alone. Practicing the highest-quality medicine, even at a sacrifice in profit, would be an example of such an objective.

# The Target-Income Model

One popular alternative to the notion that doctors are interested only in maximizing the net income from their Medicare practice is to suppose that doctors have a target income, rather than the maximum possible income, as an objective. The simple version of this theory suggests that there is some fixed number of dollars, given time and effort, to which a doctor aspires. Although this simple approach is useful as a first approximation, it has some obvious logical problems. One problem is that the explanation implies that doctors will do anything to make more money if they expect their income to be below the target, but that they are not attracted at all by the prospect of extra money once their income hits the target (McGuire and Pauly 1991). But human beings are unlikely to make such a leap in ascribing value. That is, it seems implausible that a person would do nothing to raise income above the target yet would do anything to keep income from falling below the target.

The other logical problem is that the simple target-income theory is incomplete; it is incapable of answering certain crucial questions. For example, suppose a doctor is forced to accept a lower price for one of the services he or she sells. The target-income model says that volume will be increased to make up for the lost income. Will the increase in volume be in the service with the price cut, on all other services, or on some other specific services that are highly profitable? The simple target-income model does not enlighten us.

## The sophisticated model

To solve these problems, analysts have been developing a more sophisticated version of the notion of target income (Evans 1974; Pauly 1980; McGuire and Pauly 1991). This version solves the problems just discussed by proposing that there is a trade-off for the doctor when he or she acts to raise income. The idea is that there are some services that the doctor knows are most appropriate in certain situations and that patients would demand if given accurate, complete, and perfectly truthful advice. (The advice depends, of course, on what the doctor knows, which is usually much less than is needed for absolute certainty.) The doctor probably will receive some positive income if this advice is given or this ideal quantity is provided, but even more income could be generated if the doctor induces or creates demand for services beyond those warranted by the "full truth." As we showed earlier, if only money matters to the doctor, he or she will always induce the maximum amount of demand. It is plausible, however, that the doctor suffers a kind of psychic cost from deviating from his or her "heart of hearts" belief in the best form of therapy or the best level of advice. There is, after all, sufficient uncertainty and ambiguity in knowledge about the effectiveness of care to justify more service-intensive types of care, especially if these services do not put the patient at much more risk and only take the patient's time or Medicare's money. But at some point this justification becomes somewhat more difficult.

The sophisticated target-income model assumes, therefore, that a kind of "cost of conscience" exists in creating demand. It is a cost that at least some doctors are sometimes willing to pay to enhance income a little, but ultimately it limits their willingness to induce demand. Some doctors probably increase their income by providing a style of care that is more intensive than they feel perfectly comfortable with but that they judge to be not unreasonable, given the reward.

We have just argued that the physician would be inducing demand only if he or she creates demand beyond what is needed based on fully truthful advice. But consider the situation in which the patient desires a level of services below what the physician believes would maximize health, so that a gap would occur between what the patient believes he or she needs and what the doctor would provide had he or she been allowed to act beyond the patient's wishes (independent of any effects on income). For now, assume the doctor would not provide additional information that would convince the patient that more care would be beneficial, because the time and effort required to convince the patient would be more costly to the physician than the additional revenue would justify. If the physician found, however, that an economic reason existed for changing the amount of information provided to the patient (e.g., an increase in price or a decrease in the resources required to convince the patient), then he or she might provide information to the patient in the hope of narrowing the gap between what the patient desires and what the physician believes would be beneficial to the patient.

Another consideration is that the doctor may not experience a psychic cost for increasing the amount of services recommended to the patient, if charging a higher price for a service changed the physician's interpretation of the literature about services for which indications are uncertain or ambiguous. This implies that the "heart of hearts" belief that guides the doctor in choosing the best form of therapy or the best level of advice is not fixed and might be influenced by messages the physician draws from the payment scheme. It could even be argued that society's message to the physician about what it values is implicit in the price it is willing to pay for services.

## Determinants of inducement

The critical idea here is that changes in the level of volume brought about by changes in the level of inducement can be best understood by looking at the trade-off between money income and psychic comfort. For example, if the price of one service were raised considerably, this explanation says that the doctor would be sorely tempted to induce more demand, because the psychic cost would be the same as before but the reward would be greater. The theory also says, however, that the doctor would not recommend more profitable services without limit, because his or her ethical sense would (eventually) be offended by trying to encourage use by patients who do not stand to get much benefit from the service.

Finally, this model notes that the change in the trade-off really depends on two considerations that point in opposite directions: the "marginal net-income reward" just discussed and the value the doctor attaches to being able to practice ideal medicine. The value of practicing ideal medicine may itself be affected by the doctor's income. When doctors' incomes are low, with heavy obligations and high fixed costs, they might put less value on practicing medicine in an ideal way than if a windfall should dramatically raise their incomes. This notion helps to build a case for the existence of target-income behavior. Specifically, suppose the prices of all the services a doctor provides to Medicare patients were cut. Income would be reduced. It might not be surprising, therefore, to see additional inducement of demand for all services (not necessarily in a uniform pattern, however) because the doctor feels an increased need for the money, even though the profit from doing so is less. Indeed, the relative strength of the "marginal reward" effect, relative to the effect of having a lower income, determines whether the volume response to a price cut is positive or negative (McGuire and Pauly 1991).

## The Patient Agency Model

The third model of behavior does not rely on direct economic explanations of physician behavior, in spite of the fact that much of the relevant economics literature emphasizes physicians' responsiveness to changes in the price paid for their services. The patient agency model suggests that physicians seek primarily to serve as their patients' agents. A substantial portion of the physician's satisfaction with practice is fulfilled by serving successfully as the patient's advocate. In this role, the physician makes decisions that represent what is or is perceived to be in the patient's best interest. As the patient's agent, the physician makes decisions that are believed to be the decisions the patient would make if the patient had as much information as the physician. Like profit maximization, this model serves as a benchmark for purposes of predicting price effects on volume and intensity.

There are several components to this model of medical decision making (Eisenberg 1986). First, the physician's primary role as healer demands that he or she attempt to optimize the patient's clinical outcomes, given the level of technology available. Second, the physician also will want to serve as the patient's economic agent, trying to make decisions about the use of medical services while keeping in mind the financial impact on the patient. Third, doctors will be influenced by their patients' health preferences, which are manifest in patients' demands for medical care. Finally, convenience and other patient preferences will influence the decisions of physicians who are attempting to act in their patients' best interests.

## Models of patient agency behavior

The general concept of the physician as the patient's agent is reasonably clear, and one implication of this model, in contrast to the other two models, is immediately obvious: there will be no inducement if the doctor acts as the patient's perfect agent. Ambuiguity arises, however, in connection with the doctor's pricing of the services rendered, since this is the basis of the doctor's net income. To begin to clarify this ambiguity, we can differentiate six submodels of agency behavior based on six types of agents: the altruistic agent, the market agent, the competitive agent, the social agent, the clinical agent, and the economic agent.

The *altruistic agent* acts in the best interest of his or her patient. If there is a medical service, provided by the physician-agent or someone else, that would provide medical benefit to the patient but for which the patient is unable or unwilling to pay, the physician should set the price of his or her own services sufficiently low enough that the patient would be willing to buy the needed service. This model implies that the doctor would provide beneficial services at prices well below cost to patients who felt they could not afford them; and some patients would receive free care.

This model does not seem useful as an analytic tool (although some physicians surely are altruistic in this sense). The average price of the physician-agent's own services must always be at least enough to cover cost, whatever that may mean. Although there may be instances when the physician offers charity care, in whole or in part, these must be the exception and not the rule if the otherwise unsubsidized physician is to remain in practice.

The *market agent* sets the price for services he or she provides at the net-income (profit) maximizing price, and chooses as the quantity of those services the amount the patient would have preferred at that price if he or she were fully informed. That is, the physician-agent calculates what price he or she would be able to charge in a market with fully informed patients, but with less than perfect competition because of monopolies or monopolistic competition elements in the market.

The *competitive agent* chooses quantities of *other* providers' services in the same way that market agents choose them (i.e., basing the choice on the fully informed patient's preference). But the competitive physician-agent prices his or her *own* services at what would have been the competitive price. The difference between this model and the preceding one is that, in the market model, the physician may price services above cost and achieve whatever monopoly prices would have been obtainable in some (hypothetical) fully informed but less than perfectly competitive market. Under this competitive model, the physician sets price at cost, including both the cost of practice inputs and some measure of the opportunity cost of his or her own time.

The ambiguity here is obvious: if the physician needs to act as an agent, there must have been enough imperfect patient information in the market to permit the physician to charge a price above the competitive level. If a physician wishes nevertheless to act as the patient's agent, which price should be assigned to his or her services? It is probably not as high a price as would prevail in a market with inducement, but it is not obvious that it should be the competitive price either.

Of course, if Medicare should set the price the physician may receive, this ambiguity is cleared up because the price is given. In practice, however, Medicare sets a maximum price, and the doctor would provide benefit to the patient from charging less than that price. As the new Medicare physician payment law gradually reduces the maximum price the physician can achieve under balance billing to a figure closer to what Medicare uses as the basis for its reimbursement, this problem becomes less important.

The *social agent* is one who wishes to maximize the welfare of all individuals in society, given the desires people have for goods other than health care and given limited resources. In all the agent models discussed previously, the quantity of services the physician chooses equals the quantity the patient would desire given the patient's insurance coverage—that is, given the patient's level of out-of-pocket payment. Even if the gross price that providers receive is set equal to (opportunity) cost, the quantity of services the patient would desire is greater than the quantity that represents an appropriate trade-off between costs and benefits. The patient who pays only 20 percent of the cost of physician services will, when given correct information, seek care so long as the benefit is greater than 20 percent of the cost. The question is whether the physician acting as agent should advise the patient to seek this level of care. It represents a level that is best for the individual patient, but inferior from the viewpoint of society (or all consumers or taxpayers taken together). Is the physician who wishes to act as a perfect agent supposed to be the agent of the individual patient (or small subset of all patients), or is he or she supposed to be a social agent, acting on behalf of all actual and potential patients?

Discussions of patient agency models of physician behavior have not been able to resolve this conundrum. At present, perhaps the most useful thing that can be said is that the physician who would want to act as an agent for society might find such behavior infeasible because of uncertainty about what society would want, and because he or she might not attract any patients if service use were constrained to the cost-beneficial level.

The *clinical agent* is motivated by an interest in improving the health of his or her patients. Physicians' concern for their patients' health has been shown to be a major determinant of utilization patterns (Eisenberg 1986). Physicians' principal professional motivation is to apply their knowledge and ability to improving or maintaining the health of persons who have turned to them for help. The hypothesis behind this model of behavior is that, once the physician has agreed to treat a patient, he or she derives a sense of personal utility from the patient's health, and this motivation overrides concern for the financial welfare of either the physician or the patient.

Clinicians who write about differences in physician utilization assume that a doctor would want to give better care if he or she knew what that better care was (Eisenberg 1986). Medical decision making involves substantial uncertainty, however, and the strategy that would promote patient health is not always clear. This uncertainty may exist because data are not available, because the data are available but not known to the physician making the decision, or because the available data cannot be processed effectively. The reasons for deficiencies in a practicing physician's knowledge are many, but the psychic and financial costs of acquiring new information are two important factors that influence the physician's ability to reduce uncertainty.

Given this uncertainty, in any particular patient-doctor encounter it is not surprising that physicians seeking to provide optimal care are influenced by forces outside the immediate doctor–patient interaction. In particular, the doctor's knowledge or opinion of what constitutes best care will influence his or her action. When there is uncertainty about indications, procedures, or protocols, variations in decisions about what constitutes best care are likely. Given this scenario, physicians' decisions can be changed if physicians are provided with better, or more authoritative, advice about appropriate treatment methods. Changing the price the doctor gets, in this model, will not influence variations in practice patterns, but changing information on standards will.

The *economic agent* acts out of concern for the patient's financial status. In addition to the influence of objective information, as well as the recommendations and advice of peers and professional leaders, the physician-agent is influenced by financial considerations from the perspective of their impact on the patient's well-being. Evidence does indeed suggest that physicians are sensitive to the financial impact of medical care on their patients (Eisenberg 1986; Eisenberg and Williams 1981; Long, Cummings, and Frisof 1983; Hoey et al. 1982; Cohen et al. 1982), even though this effect may be smaller than those concerned with cost containment would desire. Despite their generally poor knowledge of medical care prices, patients' insurance coverage, and patients' financial status, physicians do seem to respond to the cost of care to their patients. Some evidence (e.g., based on patient- versus physician-initiated visits, use of laboratory tests, and hospitalization) suggests that the demand for medical care is influenced more by physicians' decisions on behalf of patients than by patients' own decisions (Eisenberg 1986).

**Patient preferences and demand**

Patient demand for medical services is a manifestation of several factors, including user price, convenience, perceived value, and alternative sources of relief. As the patient's agent, the physician will want to consider these factors in choosing the appropriate clinical strategy. Perhaps most difficult for the physician is understanding the patient's preferences, or utilities, for various health states. Because patients may find it difficult to articulate their preferences, and physicians may find it difficult to discuss their patients' values, physician decisions on behalf of patients may be misguided. If a physician attempts to serve as the patient's agent but does not understand the patient's utilities, it is possible that the patient's preference will be misrepresented during the physician's decision-making process. If better information about patient values, and about costs, could be communicated to the doctor-as-agent, decisions about volume and intensity often would change.

**Patient convenience**

Convenience for the patient also may influence utilization patterns under the patient agency model. For example, patients may prefer to have laboratory tests drawn by their own physician rather than going elsewhere for venipuncture. Economic factors inevitably interact with the desire for convenience. Although patients who travel farther for laboratory testing may find lower prices, they also incur greater travel costs and greater opportunity costs in doing so.

## Other factors

The behavioral elements of medical decision making discussed in this chapter focus on the role of the physician as the patient's agent and the physician's financial considerations. Yet physician behavior is also determined by the physician's own role in the profession and his or her personal preferences. The powerful influence of professional leadership has profound implications for peer review and educational influence (Eisenberg 1986). Physicians' decisions are influenced by their desire to employ a particular style of practice, their personal characteristics, and the practice setting. In addition, the desire to serve the social good is a noneconomic behavioral motivation that needs to be considered in predicting or understanding physicians' responses to changes in the medical care system, particularly those designed to influence their behavior.

## References

Cohen, D. I., P. Jones, B. Littenberg, and D. Neuhauser. 1982. "Does Cost Information Availability Reduce Physician Test Usage? A Randomized Clinical Trial with Unexpected Results." *Medical Care* 20: 286–92.

Eisenberg, J. M. 1986. *Doctors' Decisions and the Cost of Medical Care*. Ann Arbor, MI: Health Administration Press.

Eisenberg, J. M., and S. V. Williams. 1981. "Cost Containment and Changing Physicians' Practice Behavior: Can the Fox Learn to Guard the Chicken Coop?" *Journal of the American Medical Association* 246: 2195–2201.

Evans, R. 1974. "Supplier-Induced Demand: Some Empirical Evidence and Implications." In *The Economics of Health*, edited by M. Perlman, 162–73. New York: Macmillan.

Hoey, J., J. M. Eisenberg, W. O. Spitzer, and D. Thomas. 1982. "Physician Sensitivity to the Price of Diagnostic Tests: A U.S.–Canadian Analysis." *Medical Care* 20: 302–7.

Long, M. J., K. M. Cummings, and K. B. Frisof. 1983. "The Role of Perceived Price in Physicians' Demand for Diagnostic Tests." *Medical Care* 21: 243–50.

McGuire, T. G., and M. V. Pauly. 1991. "Physician Response to Fee Changes with Multiple Payers." *Journal of Health Economics* 10: 385–410.

Pauly, M. V. 1980. *Doctors and Their Workshops*. Chicago: National Bureau of Economic Research, The University of Chicago Press.

Zuckerman, S., W. P. Welch, and G. C. Pope. 1988. *A Geographic Index of Physician Practice Costs*. Working Paper 3710-04-02. Washington, DC: The Urban Institute.

Part **II**

# Analysis of Controls

# Introduction to Part II

The chapters in this part of the book focus on various controls on the volume of physician services and their potential effects on health care costs, quality, and availability. Before discussing these anticipated effects, it is important to consider some issues regarding volume control in general.

First, any attempt to control Medicare Part B volume would require an explicit decision about whether the control would be mandatory for all physicians and all beneficiaries, or whether certain groups could "opt out" in return for lower unit prices or some other concession. A determination concerning whether or not to allow balance billing would need to be part of this decision. It may be reasonable to allow individuals to pay for additional services with their own funds, but the implications for the particular control and its overall effectiveness of allowing physicians and beneficiaries to opt out should be considered beforehand.

There is an implicit trade-off in making this decision. Using mandatory assignment would induce or compel some doctors to accept the lower Medicare price, as well as restrictions on balance billing, rather than forgo Medicare patients. The beneficiaries who use these doctors, and the Medicare program, would presumably be better off. But some doctors may refuse to accept assignment, and Medicare beneficiaries who would have used them are worse off, the more so because the beneficiaries are not even permitted to volunteer to pay to supplement what Medicare pays in order to get a preferred doctor. Some beneficiaries will benefit, others will be harmed. It is difficult to say whether the average beneficiary will win or lose, or even whether the well-being of the average beneficiary is a relevant measure of desirability. The answer may depend in part on whether or not the higher prices that mandatory assignment prohibits are thought to yield monopoly returns (i.e., profits in excess of what a competitive market would allow).

Second, the controls discussed in Chapters 4–10 need not be implemented in isolation; combinations may be more effective. Clinical guidelines, for example, would be a useful adjunct to any other volume control. Likewise, rigorous outpatient utilization review could be implemented along with expenditure caps or changes in copayments so as to monitor the appropriateness of services provided. One of the major reasons for considering collapsed procedure coding as a control is that it would enable closer monitoring of "upcoding" (the practice of assigning a more complex code than is appropriate); in this case, expanded utilization review would be necessary for effectiveness. Other techniques could be used with the controls as well. Case management, for example, could readily be used in conjunction with utilization review, and capitation could be used with the current or a modified version of copayment or under an expenditure cap. Thus, although seven controls are analyzed separately here, possible combinations should be kept in mind.

Third, any relationship between controls on the volume of physician services and inpatient volume and expenditures will have to be monitored if there is ever to be stabilization or reduction in overall health care costs. There is little sense in an approach that merely shifts costs from one site to another. Efforts should be taken to avoid inappropriate changes in the locus of care and attendant increases in overall costs. Long-term effects on health care professionals are also a consideration. The degree to which volume controls discourage entry into the medical profession in general or into individual specialties is an important factor and needs to be examined.

Finally, the widespread implementation of any of these controls should be preceded by demonstration projects. The predictions in these chapters about what is likely to happen with each control are based on thoughts about how physicians, and to a lesser extent patients, respond. However, very little empirical evidence exists to substantiate these predictions. Further, a variety of design issues bear on the ultimate effects of each control; the final form a control takes will therefore influence these effects. Demonstration projects would help to predict these more accurately and avoid or minimize adverse consequences.

Chapter 4

# Copayment

Copayment refers to cost sharing, by the beneficiary, of a portion of his or her medical bills for services covered by an insurance plan. Two of the forms of copayment that can be used to affect the volume of physician services are deductibles and coinsurance. A deductible is a set amount of out-of-pocket expenditures a patient must pay for covered services over a given time before his or her insurance begins to pay for services. In most insurance plans, including Medicare's Part B, the insured must pay a predetermined dollar amount in any given year before the insurance plan pays anything. Once the deductible is met, the beneficiary might still be responsible for paying a second kind of copayment: coinsurance. Coinsurance refers to patient responsibility for paying a percentage of the total charges in excess of the deductible. Any given insurance plan could use either, both, or neither of these forms of copayment.

This chapter offers a review of the rationale for the use of copayment as a volume and intensity control, and an explanation of how copayment is used as a control. The chapter outlines ways in which copayments can be used more effectively, with special focus on their use in the Medicare program. Finally, the chapter explores the probable effectiveness of copayment as a control on the volume and intensity of physican services, based on empirical evidence and what theory suggests.

## Rationale for the Use of Copayment

There is strong empirical evidence that larger out-of-pocket payments are associated with lower total volumes of and expenditures on physician services (Newhouse et al. 1981). The evidence of this effect is discussed later in this chapter. Compared to a situation in which the consumer pays nothing out-of-pocket, deductibles and coinsurance can reduce total spending by a substantial amount. Without a system of self-responsibility in which beneficiaries pay some part of the cost of care, patients will seek all care they believe promises some potential benefit, no matter how slight the benefit and no matter how high the cost. This behavior—using more services when insurance covers them—is known as a "moral hazard" in insurance theory, and it may occur whenever the patient does not pay the full cost of services received. At the same time, physicians who are paid a sufficiently high fee per unit of service will be willing to provide such care, no matter what behavioral model governs their response—profit maximization, target income, or market-type patient agency, although their response will be tempered in the target-income model if income has exceeded the target. Volume increases would not occur if the physician acted as a social agent.

The thought that copayments could help to limit cost and reduce services was presumably what motivated Congress to require a deductible and 20 percent copayment for most Medicare Part B services. Despite the presence of this feature, however, Part B expenditures have grown at a rapid rate. Such growth does not necessarily mean that copayment itself (or other cost-control devices) is ineffective. It may be that copayment keeps expenditures lower than they would be otherwise, but that other incentives or influences drive costs upward.

In the private sector, the use of copayments as a control on the volume of physician services would be straightforward: if volume is regarded as excessive, simply increasing the amount of either the deductible or the coinsurance or both would be expected to decrease the demand for services. The major concern for private insurance companies using this tactic would be to remain competitive with other plans so as not to lose business. Similarly, corporations and businesses that provide health insurance as an employee benefit would need to exercise caution in offering a plan that has unusually high copayments, because they need to compete with other firms for workers. If, however, an increment in cost sharing could be found that was consistent with continued competition in the labor market, the use of this approach to restrain the volume and intensity of physician services would be relatively simple.

Within the Medicare program, following a similar approach is somewhat more complicated. Two factors unique to Medicare make increments in copayments more difficult to achieve and less effective (relative to private insurance plans) if they are achieved. First, the political nature of the Medicare program makes a potential policy change regarding copayments controversial. Raising copayments (or heightening their impact) lessens the value of the program to the elderly and amounts to a cut in their benefits. Given the political strength of this demographic group, legislators tend to shy away from such proposals. Cash transfers to beneficiaries could compensate for increased copayments, but this too is probably politically difficult, if not infeasible.

Second, even if such a policy could be enacted, it would be less effective than expected as a volume control within Medicare because of the role of Medigap policies, the private insurance plans purchased by Medicare beneficiaries that pay for much of the copayment amount. Approximately 70 percent of Medicare Part B enrollees either purchase such policies or receive similar protection from out-of-pocket expenses through simultaneous enrollment in Medicaid. Although Medigap purchasers as a group may pay at least as much in premiums as they would with higher copayments, without such policies Medigap insurance dissociates the cost of care from the actual receipt of services by the individual Medicare beneficiary, thereby lessening the disincentives copayments are intended to provide.

Because of these complicating factors in the Medicare market and the relative simplicity of the private insurance market, at least with respect to copayments, this chapter is focused on the implications for the Medicare program of this approach to volume control.

## Copayment as a Control on Volume in Medicare

Copayment is the most extensively used health services utilization control in the United States. With the exception of capitation arrangements, copayments are used by virtually every type of health insurance plan, including Medicare. Medicare Part B beneficiaries must meet a $100 deductible per year (effective 1991) and then are responsible for 20 percent coinsurance on Medicare-allowed charges for most outpatient and physician services (PPRC 1990). There is also a Part A deductible (currently $652 per benefit period) and some Part A coinsurance on long hospital stays. Copayment arrangements vary among private health insurance plans, but typically they are of the same general form. One important difference is that most private insurance also limits the total amount of out-of-pocket payments through a stop-loss feature; Medicare (since the repeal of catastrophic coverage) does not.

The use of copayment as a strategy to control the growth of Medicare Part B payments appears on the surface to be less politically attractive than some other options. In contrast to volume-control schemes in which the burden is initially placed on providers, in this strategy the burden is placed directly on retirees. Given the relatively high average level of income in elderly households, sharing some of the burden with the nonpoor elderly would not be obviously inequitable, but it is sure to be unpopular. On the other hand, of all the volume-limiting strategies, copayment provides the most unambiguous empirical evidence of effectiveness. It also appears to have the greatest magnitude of effectiveness. Evidence suggests that the effect of copayment on expenditure is nearly twice as great as the effect of capitation.

How then could third party payers such as Medicare make better use of copayments? The most obvious way of using copayments to produce further reductions in overall medical care service use and payer expenditures would simply be to increase the level of copayments. Despite the possibility of offsetting increases in the purchase of Medigap coverage, this would probably reduce Part B spending substantially. Taylor et al. (1988) estimate, for example, that an increase in the Part B copayment from 20 percent to 25 percent could reduce Medicare outlays by as much as 11 percent. Because the decline in outlays is less than the decline in coverage, raising copayments must result in a decrease in total volume and intensity, as well as in Medicare's share of the payments.

The disadvantage of increasing copayment is that requiring the patient to pay more will increase beneficiary exposure to financial risk and reduce the value of Medicare benefits. For some beneficiaries, bearing this higher cost would be difficult and might deter them from seeking appropriate services. Are there alternative, less objectionable ways of redesigning the Medicare program to make better use of copayments?

## Making existing Medicare copayments more effective

The growth of Medigap coverage over the years has meant that the real out-of-pocket unit price for Part B services has not increased very much, even though real medical costs have increased rapidly. Medigap coverage insulates most Medicare beneficiaries from the effect of increases in the cost of medical care, despite the intent of the framers of the Medicare program to use copayments to enlist beneficiaries in the fight to keep expenditures down.

To be sure, not all elderly persons buy private Medigap coverage. Elderly with very low incomes have their copayments covered by Medicaid. Private Medigap coverage, in contrast, is positively related to income or wealth. The well-to-do elderly are almost entirely covered, whereas those beneficiaries just slightly above the Medicaid eligibility maximum are least likely to have Medigap coverage and most likely to be subject to out-of-pocket payments. This arrangement seems less than equitable; it stems in part from the all-or-nothing nature of Medicaid and in part from the fact that insurance coverage is generally a normal good—one for which purchases increase as income rises. Thus, simply increasing copayments, although it would deter Medicare expenditures, would have a negative effect on low-income elderly.

It might be argued that the relatively low-income elderly would be most responsive to out-of-pocket payments in any case, so that the current pattern of coverage, given that at least 70 percent would have Medigap coverage, is most conducive to constraining expenditures. However, it is also possible that the low-income elderly, deterred from using Part B services by uninsured copayments, would put off care that would prevent more serious, and more expensive, illness. In the RAND Health Insurance Experiment, for example, enrollees in cost-sharing plans used fewer preventive services than enrollees in capitated plans, although there were no attributable negative effects on health and no relationship to income as a result (Manning et al. 1984, 1987). At the same time, it is likely that the services of low marginal value that purportedly have fed the growth in Part B expenditures tend to be concentrated more among the high-income elderly who have Medigap coverage.

For those persons who do buy Medigap coverage, increased Medicare copayments presumably do not affect the volume of services demanded; they simply raise Medigap premiums. The situation is, in a sense, the worst of all worlds. Copayments do not serve their intended function of controlling volume and expenditures because they are rendered ineffective by private coverage. But the coverage itself, because it is often sold as individual coverage rather than as group coverage, has a very high administrative cost, often as much as 50 percent of Medigap premiums. Were it not for the equity consequences, efficiency would be improved and administrative cost lowered by abolishing Medicare copayments for high-income elderly (thereby eliminating the need for Medigap policies), because Medicare could surely provide complete coverage at lower administrative cost. In short, the current situation is one in which Medicare copayments do not deter expenditure but do add to the cost of paper shuffling, which society has to bear.

The implication of using cost sharing to control Medicare volume and intensity is clear. Before copayments are raised and Medicare Part B coverage is reduced, we should try to limit the extent to which the incentive effects of copayments are blunted by the purchase of Medigap coverage. This effort should be concentrated on higher-income elderly to preserve equity, and should not lead to inappropriate deterrence of use.

## Making Medigap coverage more efficient

Bringing considerations of equity and appropriateness into the policy process immediately raises the question of social objectives. If one's only objective were to cut Part B spending, simply prohibiting Medigap coverage (e.g., by denying any Medicare benefits to those who buy it) would be an effective way to do so. But it is obvious that beneficiaries who buy Medigap coverage get some benefits from it, benefits that would be lost if coverage were forbidden. To develop an appropriate policy, we should investigate the determinants of Medigap purchase and ask whether those purchases represent efficient market choices.

Research on this subject strongly suggests that current levels of purchase are probably excessive. The reason is that there are at least two strong implicit public subsidies to Medigap coverage (they are described later). Not only do these subsidies presumably lead to the purchase of Medigap coverage (which, at the margin, costs more than the benefits it provides), but these subsidies also offer larger benefits, on average, to higher-income people. Thus, both equity and efficiency could be improved by reducing or eliminating these subsidies. Elimination of the subsidies for Medigap insurance would lead not only to a reduction in the seemingly wasteful resources devoted to administering private and public insurance, but also to a decrease in Part B expenditures. Moreover, in contrast to the price-based or incentive-based volume controls, this strategy does not suffer from empirical or theoretical ambiguity as to the direction of outcome. Eliminating subsidies to Medigap policies will reduce Medigap purchases, and reduced Medigap coverage will reduce Medicare volume and cost. The magnitude of the reduction in Medicare expenditures is not certain, but there are reasons to believe that the amount could be substantial.

How is Medigap subsidized by the public? One of the subsidies actually comes from Medicare itself. Consider the consequences to Medicare's total spending if a person decides to buy Medigap coverage. If the person buys the coverage, the user price of care falls to zero, and total use of medical services rises. Some of this additional use is covered by the Medigap insurer and is built into the Medigap premium. If, however, use of services increases as a result of copayment coverage by the Medigap policy, about 80 percent of the cost of the additional Part B use is covered by Medicare, and even more of the accompanying Part A expenditures are covered. There is no mechanism to translate the message of this increased cost back to the individual purchaser of Medigap coverage.

Ideal insurance coverage, in any market, should reflect a trade-off between the benefits of risk reduction and the total cost of the increased expenditure induced by that coverage. The Medigap purchaser sees only 20 percent of the true cost of the additional use that is induced by buying Medigap coverage; the other 80 percent is simply absorbed by Medicare. In other words, all of the benefits of additional risk reduction and the value of the additional medical services whose consumption is induced are received completely by the Medigap purchaser, who pays only a fraction of their cost. Even if the risk reduction benefits are only of marginal value, and even if the benefits of additional medical care are minimal, the person may still choose the Medigap coverage.

Only Medicare's insurance operates in this fashion. In conventional private insurance markets, sellers of basic coverage (usually in a group setting) will recognize the need to raise premiums for that coverage if supplementary coverage is added. Buyers ordinarily buy all coverage from the same insurer, so this additional premium automatically gets built into the premium for a policy of greater coverage. However, Medicare does not take account of the purchase of important supplemental coverage, failing to adjust its own premium for basic Part B coverage when Medigap coverage is bought. Of course, if the buyer of supplemental coverage can keep that fact a secret from the basic insurer, no premium adjustment will be made. Private-sector "coordination of benefits" provisions exist in part to prevent this from happening.

It is easy to see how to deal with the problem of the Medicare subsidy. For those who buy Medigap coverage, the Part B premium should be adjusted upward to reflect the higher values of expected claims. The average increase in premiums that would be paid could be substantial. Taylor et al. (1988) estimate that Medicare benefits are on average 39 percent higher for those who buy a typical Medigap policy than for those who do not. Therefore, unless there is evidence that the size of this effect varies with other characteristics of the beneficiary or the policy, and assuming that this impact on expenditures is consistent across Parts A and B, an efficient program would be one that imposes a surcharge on the Part B premium of 39 percent for those who buy Medigap.

If a Medigap policy, provided individually or in an employment group, were able to demonstrate effective cost containment, then this surcharge might be reduced. But, in general, such a surcharge would improve efficiency of the health insurance scheme. Regardless of the effect on the purchase of Medigap coverage, additional surcharge revenues would help to offset rising Part B costs.

As noted, the likelihood of buying Medigap coverage is strongly related to beneficiary income or wealth. Therefore, the Medigap subsidy that Medicare pays provides benefits that actually increase as income increases. On average, equity would also be improved by increasing Part B premiums for those who buy Medigap.

For purposes of this discussion, the most important impact of this corrective measure would be an expected decline in the number of persons who buy Medigap coverage. If a person decides to forgo Medigap coverage when faced with a larger net premium (i.e., the Medigap premium plus a surcharge on the Part B premium) that reflects the true additional expense caused by that coverage, it must be because, in truth, the benefits from that Medigap coverage are not worth their cost. Consequently, society is made better off if no purchase occurs, because the value of the resources saved is greater than the value of the benefits lost. Because many allege that Medigap purchasers are more likely to overestimate the value of such coverage, imperfect consumer information will not offset this conclusion.

The other subsidy to Medigap coverage is paid to those whose coverage is furnished by their former employer as part of postretirement health benefits. We refer here to benefits for retirees who are also eligible for Medicare, not to benefits for early retirees. Employers' payments for such group Medigap coverage is a tax-deductible expense for the employer, but it is not counted as part of the retiree's taxable income. In contrast, elderly persons who do not have employer-provided coverage must pay for their Medigap coverage out of their income, at least some of which is taxable.

Here again, the tax subsidy is greatest to higher-income retirees, both because their employers are more likely to provide coverage and because the taxes they avoid are collected at a higher rate. It is true that employer-provided payments for Medigap coverage are not treated as favorably for tax purposes as employer payments for pensions or annuities, because in the latter case employers can shield from taxation the interest accumulated on prefunded amounts. However, in contrast to the treatment of pensions in which the income from the tax-shielded contributions is treated as taxable income when received by the retiree, Medigap benefits are not treated as part of taxable income at any time.

With the recent publication by the Financial Accounting Standards Board of new accounting rules concerning postretirement benefits, employer-provided Medigap benefits may be somewhat restricted in any case, although there is as yet little evidence of substantial cutbacks (Coopers & Lybrand 1991). There may be a basis for preserving the tax subsidy to employer-provided benefits to early retirees if we wish to preserve neutral incentives for such retirement. But there is no obvious case for subsidizing Medigap benefits, given the presumption that the current level of Medicare benefits is an adequate representation of social concern for the level of insurance coverage that elderly people should have.

The solution to this dilemma is to reduce the tax subsidy. This could be done by taxing the value of employer-provided Medigap coverage as part of the retiree's income. Such a strategy would make the Medigap benefits less attractive for all workers. The higher the expected incomes of a firm's workers, the greater the elimination of tax subsidy; and this should discourage purchase of inefficient coverage.

It would be possible to achieve greater equity by treating subsidies for Medigap coverage differently for different elderly households with different incomes. Elderly persons whose incomes are close to the poverty line might be exempt from the surcharge on the Part B premium should they choose to purchase Medigap, and they might be permitted to receive tax-free employer-provided benefits. Either of these subsidies could decline as income rises. But the high-income elderly, say the 25 percent of the elderly who have family incomes in excess of $25,000, might appropriately be subject to the tax and the removal of the tax subsidy.

Still another modification might be to permit Medigap to be untaxed, and to allow group coverage to remain tax-free, for Medigap benefits that do not reduce the impact of current Part B copayments. Medigap coverage for nursing home care, for example, could be permitted without triggering a Part B surcharge. If we reduce the subsidy for inappropriate Medigap coverage but continue it for what is regarded as more appropriate coverage, even current subsidy recipients need not be penalized financially.

It is obvious that public policy has been of two minds about Part B copayments and Medigap coverage. The argument that copayments help to deter use of services of marginal value is presumably the basis for including copayments in Part B coverage. And yet, Medigap coverage has been treated in ways that actually diminish the amount of cost sharing. In fact, the Baucus Amendment (Section 507 of the Social Security Amendments of 1980) sets forth new standards for Medigap policies that *require* policies to cover all coinsurance (Cafferata 1985).

The reason for the ambivalence of public policy on coinsurance for Medicare is probably the fear that the service utilization discouraged by copayments may sometimes be appropriate utilization. There is some evidence that copayment may reduce the use of both appropriate and inappropriate services. In practice, however, other control devices run the same risks. Changing physician prices, limiting use by utilization review, or moving toward capitation can also lead to mistakes. Even imperfect guidelines may do harm as well as good. The question, then, is whether increased copayment would be more likely than other alternatives of equal effectiveness to discourage appropriate use when applied in actual (rather than idealized) settings.

There are other factors to consider about the possibility of inappropriate deterrence. First, even if the financial incentives to patients push them toward using fewer services, physicians face countervailing incentives to encourage use, which they can do by offering accurate, but persuasive, information about the benefits of care. Second, copayments already are used in the Medicare program; hence, it is inconsistent public policy to employ copayments and at the same time to assert that they discourage appropriate use and therefore should not be strengthened. If copayments do that much damage, they should be abolished for everyone, not (in effect) just for those who can afford Medigap coverage. Finally, it would be possible, at some administrative cost, to waive copayments for certain types of services that tend to be underused, if such services can be identified.

Because only a few Medigap policies cover any balance-billed amounts, this discussion is limited to Medigap coverage of copayments. To the extent, however, that reduction in Medigap coverage would lead to less coverage of balance-billed amounts, Part B volume and intensity would be further reduced. Moreover, because high-income persons are more likely to buy Medigap coverage, discouraging such coverage would actually be a step toward equalizing access to those physicians who do not accept assignment.

## Effectiveness of Copayment as a Volume Control

It seems likely that these strategies to reduce the purchase of Medigap insurance would be effective and would, in turn, reduce the level of Part B volume and expenditures. Even if responses are small, additional revenues will have been raised; thus, this strategy to regenerate existing Part B copayments cannot fail to do some fiscal good for the U.S. Treasury.

There is good evidence that strengthening copayments in Medicare's Part B coverage would have a significant effect on service utilization and overall expenditures. Much of this optimism comes from the empirical evidence on copayments, which is reviewed here. The models of physician behavior also provide reason to believe that this would be the case.

### Empirical evidence

The best evidence available on the effect of beneficiary copayment on the use of services comes from the RAND Health Insurance Experiment (HIE). The study was a controlled trial of alternative health insurance policies that ranged from free care to those imposing 25 percent, 50 percent, or 95 percent coinsurance, up to a maximum dollar amount depending on participating families' incomes. Over 2,500 families and 7,700 persons from six areas of the country participated in the study for three to five years. The results of this study showed that as the extent of coinsurance for which the beneficiary is responsible falls, total expenditures on medical care rise (Newhouse et al. 1981). Averaged across all sites, expenditures per person in the 95 percent coinsurance plan were 69 percent of those in the free-care plan. Put another way, free care resulted in an increase in expenditures of nearly 50 percent.

Data from the HIE allowed for analysis of the effects of coinsurance on various components of care as well. In each site and year analyzed, expenditures on ambulatory services rose as coinsurance fell (Newhouse et al. 1981). The likelihood of hospitalization was higher in the free-care plan than in the one plan that provided inpatient care at no expense to the beneficiary (but had a 95 percent coinsurance rate for outpatient expenses). The HIE authors suggest that such an effect may occur because physicians see persons as outpatients less frequently if they are covered under such a plan and thus have fewer opportunities to hospitalize them (Newhouse et al. 1981). Overall, adults who received free care were hospitalized 31 percent more often than those in cost-sharing plans (Siu et al. 1986).

Adults who were not in cost-sharing plans used 86 percent more antibiotics in the ambulatory setting than those who were, which resulted in expenditures that were about 60 percent higher than in cost-sharing programs (Foxman et al. 1987). No difference was found in the charge per prescription under coinsurance, suggesting that the effect of cost sharing on antibiotic use comes about primarily through a reduction in visits rather than as a result of reduced prescribing per visit (Foxman et al. 1987). Overall, drug use in the ambulatory setting increased as coinsurance decreased, at a rate similar to increases in total per capita expenditures. All cost-sharing plans showed significantly lower drug expenditures than the free plan (Liebowitz, Manning, and Newhouse 1985).

Emergency services expenses were 42 percent higher for persons who were not in cost-sharing plans than for those with significant coinsurance; they were approximately 16 percent higher than for those in plans with relatively low cost sharing (O'Grady et al. 1985). Nearly all of these expenditures were caused by the decision to use any emergency services, as opposed to using greater amounts of service once emergency care was sought.

Does cost sharing selectively decrease care considered "not medically appropriate"? In a study of the appropriateness of hospitalizations of the HIE population, Siu et al. (1986) found that cost sharing decreased admissions labeled "appropriate" and "inappropriate" by equal proportions. Emergency rooms, however, were used more often for less urgent conditions in the free-care plan than in the 25 percent coinsurance plan, suggesting that some deterrence of less appropriate care may occur (O'Grady et al. 1985).

What is the effect of beneficiary copayments on health? The HIE showed evidence of negative health impacts on hypertension control and visual acuity, but not on any of a large number of other health indicators.

Whether this qualitatively modest effect on health is worth the cost saving is obviously a value judgment. At a minimum, however, targeting certain services—hypertension control, for example—to be provided free or at very low levels of cost sharing, while still using copayments for all other services, would be one way to address the concern about adverse effects on outcomes.

Because the elderly were specifically excluded from the HIE, it is not possible to generalize the results to that group. However, there was no evidence that adults' response to the level of cost sharing was influenced by age.

### Anticipated impacts on volume and intensity:
### A theoretical analysis

An increase in copayment decreases patient demand for services, not only because patients seek less care or seek it less often, but also because it is more difficult for doctors to induce demand for services. That is, if previously a physician had been able to recommend a more expensive service with virtually no resistance from the patient, then with greater cost sharing, patients are more likely to resist such recommendations. Thus, in the target-income model of physician behavior, the ability of the physician to provide marginally useful or more expensive services will be diminished. The profit-maximizing physician will not be able to do so, and the market-agent physician will not wish to offer marginal services.

Whether or not this results in an overall reduction in volume and expenditures depends on whether excess supply or excess demand previously existed in the health care market. If, for example, there had previously been a greater demand for services than physicians were able to meet (i.e, a situation of excess demand or shortage), higher copayments might have no effect on actual use or cost—the only effect would be a decline in the extent of shortage. Because there is no change in the prices doctors receive, their supply decisions do not change. Alternatively, if physicians previously had met all demand for services and still had been willing to supply more (i.e., excess supply existed), then a decrease in patient demand would result in a decrease in overall use and costs. In this case, the profit-maximizing physician would provide fewer services. The physician who targets income, however, might want to keep his or her income at the target level. To do so, he or she would need to provide more services at the same price, which might be accomplished by working harder at convincing patients that they need more service. Because excess demand does not generally seem to characterize either

Medicare or private markets, the most likely outcome is such a decline in volume. However, because the effectiveness of increased copayments as a strategy for volume and intensity control could depend on the supply of physicians, its effectiveness may be different in areas that have a relative oversupply of physicians than in those that have an undersupply.

Under the patient agency model, the situation would be somewhat more complicated. If the physician acts as the patient's economic agent in addition to being a health agent, then he or she may be reluctant to advocate a service if the patient will have to pay more. If the service is potentially useful, however, the doctor will want to recommend it. What is likely to happen is that the physician will make benefit-cost determinations for the patient on a service-by-service basis; in this case, use of some services will decrease (although the use of certain other services, if they are less costly substitutes, may increase). Overall effects on costs will depend on the mix of services that increase and decrease, and if the physician's judgment of benefit and cost are accurate, the cost-effectiveness of medical care should generally improve. Ellis and McGuire (1990) have recently proposed a model in which the actual quantity of services provided lies between that demanded and that supplied, when the two differ. Although this model has not yet been supported empirically, it would unequivocally suggest a negative effect of cost sharing on volume.

## Summary

More is known about the effectiveness of copayments than about any other device that might control volume and intensity. Copayments work to reduce volume, but it is less clear whether they slow the rate of growth in spending over the long term. Their effects on use are not perfect: both allegedly appropriate and allegedly inappropriate services appear to be limited in response to cost sharing. Compared to idealized forms of other controls, copayments may not look as good. Compared to the uncertainty about the effectiveness of other devices, however, and the possibility that they also may discourage provision of appropriate services, revitalizing copayments may be a relatively attractive option. Especially if accompanied by serious efforts at quality assurance, copayments could be a good way to limit the volume and intensity of physician services, both in the Medicare program and within private insurance plans. Equity and efficiency might be combined by linking greater assistance to lower-income elderly with a tax or penalty for the purchase of Medigap insurance by the elderly who are not poor.

# References

Cafferata, G. L. 1985. "Private Health Insurance Coverage of the Medicare Population and the Baucus Amendment." *Medical Care* 23: 1086–96.

Coopers & Lybrand. 1991. *Actuarial, Benefits & Compensation Information Release: Special Edition—Employers' Accounting for Postretirement Benefits Other than Pensions.* FASB Issues SFAS No. 106. Philadelphia: Coopers & Lybrand.

Ellis, R. P., and T. G. McGuire. 1990. "Optimal Payment Systems for Health Services." *Journal of Health Economics* 9: 375–96.

Foxman, B., R. B. Valdes, K. N. Lohr, G. A. Goldberg, J. P. Newhouse, and R. H. Brook. 1987. "The Effect of Cost Sharing on the Use of Antibiotics in Ambulatory Care: Results from a Population-based Randomized Controlled Trial. *Journal of Chronic Disease* 40: 429–37.

Liebowitz, A., W. G. Manning, and J. P. Newhouse. 1985. "The Demand for Prescription Drugs as a Function of Cost-Sharing." *Social Science and Medicine* 21: 1063–69.

Manning, W. G., A. Leibowitz, G. A. Goldberg, W. H. Rogers, and J. P. Newhouse. 1984. "A Controlled Trial of the Effect of a Prepaid Group Practice on Use of Services." *New England Journal of Medicine* 310: 1505–10.

Manning, W. G., J. P. Newhouse, N. Duan, E. B. Keeler, A. Leibowitz, and M. S. Marquis. 1987. "Health Insurance and the Demand for Medical Care: Evidence from a Randomized Experiment." *American Economic Review* 77: 251–77.

Newhouse, J. P., W. G. Manning, C. N. Morris, L. L. Orr, N. Duan, E. B. Keeler, A. Leibowitz, K. H. Marquis, M. S. Marquis, C. E. Phelps, and R. H. Brook. 1981. "Some Interim Results from a Controlled Trial of Cost Sharing in Health Insurance." *New England Journal of Medicine* 305: 1501–7.

O'Grady, K. F., W. G. Manning, J. P. Newhouse, and R. H. Brook. 1985. "The Impact of Cost Sharing on Emergency Department Use." *New England Journal of Medicine* 313: 484–90.

Physician Payment Review Commission (PPRC). 1990. *Annual Report to Congress.* Washington, DC: Physician Payment Review Commission.

Siu, A. L., F. A. Sonnenberg, W. G. Manning, G. A. Goldberg, E. S. Bloomfield, J. P. Newhouse, and R. H. Brook. 1986. "Inappropriate Use of Hospitals in a Randomized Trial of Health Insurance Plans." *New England Journal of Medicine* 315: 1259–66.

Taylor, A. K., P. F. Short, and C. M. Horgan. 1988. "Medigap Insurance: Friend or Foe in Reducing Medicare Deficits?" In *Health Care in America: The Political Economy of Hospitals and Health Insurance,* edited by H. E. Frech III. San Francisco: Pacific Research Institute for Public Policy.

# Chapter 5

# Clinical Guidelines and Professional Education

Clinical guidelines can be defined as the delineation of specific criteria for the use of a particular test or treatment. Guidelines in themselves simply specify "appropriate" treatment. They include no provision for monitoring or enforcement after dissemination, although their introduction may be accompanied by educational efforts aimed at relevant professionals and providers. The criteria that guidelines set forth may include *physiologic criteria*, that is, specific values or cutoffs for physiologic measurements; *clinical indicators*, such as symptoms or pertinent facts from the patient's clinical history; or *risk factors*, that is, patient habits or conditions that are significant enough in and of themselves to indicate the use of a test or treatment.

Clinical guidelines can be developed for two purposes: (1) to inform, educate, and guide providers (especially physicians) and (2) to control service utilization and, consequently, costs. Thus, there is both a medical-scientific component and a public policy component in most sets of guidelines. The medical-scientific component is the objective determination of the safety, efficacy, effectiveness, benefits, and risks of specific services under specific clinical conditions; these are based on the facts regarding the clinical impact of services. The policy component includes comparisons of the trade-offs of the service in question with those of other medical and nonmedical services, and evaluations of the effect of the service on costs. Based on these comparisons and evaluations, society or the payer must make the ethical and political judgments necessary to determine whether the benefits of the service are worth the costs. Some practices might be determined to meet acceptable levels of safety and efficacy, while others might be deemed less desirable because of high cost (e.g., organ transplants), the absence of an ethical and political consensus (e.g., abortion or genetic engineering), or other factors.

Guidelines can be used in a number of ways. They can, for example, become the basis for utilization review efforts to deny payment in cases in which indications for appropriate use are not met (considered in detail in Chapter 6). Likewise, they can be used to guide coverage policy within Medicare or private insurance plans. Such enforcement would be expected to increase the power of a guideline to control the volume or intensity of care. Yet it has been argued that the simple issuance of a guideline, with efforts to educate physicians about its contents, is also effective in changing practice (Wennberg 1985). If so, guidelines would be a particularly attractive approach to the problem of overprovision, in that they limit inappropriate care in an unobtrusive, nonregulatory way.

This chapter focuses on guidelines that are used primarily to encourage ideal medical practice by defining appropriate care and then communicating that definition to physicians and other providers. There is no explicit enforcement of the recommendations the guidelines contain. Rather, the guidelines constitute a public good in the form of pertinent information, the voluntary use of which should improve treatment. The hope that their use in this manner will also help to control volume rests on the idea that minimizing physician uncertainty about appropriate practice will lead to more appropriate utilization of the service in question.

After a review of the rationale for the use of guidelines and a consideration of the extent to which they are presently used, the chapter addresses some of the factors thought to influence the effectiveness of guidelines as controls on physician services. A discussion of the feasibility of developing rigorous, comprehensive guidelines is included. Finally, the chapter looks at the likelihood, given our knowledge and the predictions from behavioral and economic theory, that guidelines without enforcement would be an effective approach to the control of physician services. This assessment is based on available data as well as on behavioral and economic theory.

## Rationale for the Use of Guidelines

Modern medicine attempts to be scientifically based. Ideally, through clinical observation and scientific study, the safety, efficacy, effectiveness, benefits, and costs of services are determined and used to guide medical practice. It is not possible, however, for individual physicians to evaluate independently the impact of most clinical practices. The volume of medical literature is huge, of variable quality, widely diffused among a large number of journals in a variety of specialties, and often not clinically oriented. Consequently, much medical care is based on physicians' heuristics and habits, with the result that there is significant variation in the patterns of care.

By synthesizing all the evidence from diverse sources, guidelines regarding the appropriateness of specific services for specific groups of patients provide physicians with improved information for the care of their patients (Fletcher and Fletcher 1990). Guidelines can thus result in more informed providers, more appropriate service provision to patients, improved patient care and outcomes, and, often, reduced service volume and costs. Guidelines cannot substitute for clinical acumen, of course, and must therefore be used with care. Certain patients have special conditions or needs that cause them to be different from the "typical" case necessarily covered in a guideline (Fletcher and Fletcher 1990), and guidelines can become outdated as new technologies and research findings emerge (Dixon 1990). Nevertheless, for a substantial portion of cases, and especially for conditions for which multiple diagnostic and therapeutic approaches are possible, guidelines can assist the physician in providing the most appropriate care.

Publicized guidelines also offer the opportunity to inform patients of medical standards and to encourage them to become more active participants in and to assume more responsibility for their own care. An informed consumer can act as a check on busy practitioners, suggesting alternatives, inquiring about various management strategies, and raising issues of safety, effectiveness, functional outcome, and costs. An informed consumer can also encourage the physician to refrain from providing a service that offers little potential benefit relative to its cost, a decision that physicians may be reluctant to make on their own.

The primary appeal of guidelines is that they seek to improve the care provided, rather than simply to limit services or contain costs. Indeed, in some circumstances guidelines could even lead to increased volume (e.g., if a service has been underused). The outcome when guidelines are used can be no better than the guidelines themselves, of course; outcomes will not improve if a guideline recommends an ineffective strategy, which could happen if there is not sufficient data or experience on which to base a guideline.

## The Present Use of Guidelines

The use of clinical guidelines is fairly widespread in the United States, and guidelines have been developed by a variety of public and private groups. Perhaps the most familiar are those that guide immunization practices for children, set forth by American Academy of Pediatrics as early as 1938 (American Academy of Pediatrics 1938); the recommendations on adult immunization issued by the United States Centers for Disease Control (CDC 1989); and the Consensus Development Program guidelines of the National Institutes of Health (Jacoby 1985), which suggest optimal practices for a number of clinical conditions and technologies.

Other groups have also developed guidelines for their own purposes. Several professional societies have guidelines for practice relevant to their membership. Examples include the immunization guidelines of the American Academy of Pediatrics, as noted above; the technology-related guidelines of the American College of Physicians' Clinical Efficacy Assessment Project (White and Ball 1985); and the Diagnostic and Therapeutic Technology Assessment (DATTA) project of the American Medical Association's Council on Scientific Affairs (Woolf 1990). At least 21 other medical specialty societies have issued guidelines as well (Woolf 1990; AMA 1989).

Insurers use guidelines to inform providers of what practices will be reimbursed in a given clinical situation. An example is the Medical Necessity Project of the Blue Cross and Blue Shield Association of America (Morris 1987). Insurers also use "physician education" regarding appropriate utilization of services fairly extensively as a volume control (see the report on our survey of Medicare carriers in Appendix A). In the course of their research projects, private research groups such as RAND have developed guidelines for the use of selected medical and surgical procedures (Chassin et al. 1989). Nonprofit societies such as the American Cancer Society (1988) also issue recommendations on cancer screening and other relevant practices.

The use of carefully derived, objective guidelines appears to be widely accepted by physicians, insurers, and patients. One recent development in health services research that promises to further the use of clinical guidelines is the establishment of a national agency aimed at supporting studies of the effectiveness of various medical practices. As a new component of the U.S. Department of Health and Human Services, the Agency for Health Care Policy and Research (AHCPR) has as its major goal the improvement of the effectiveness and appropriateness of medical care through the support of research on the impact of medical care on patients' survival, health status, functional capacity, and quality of life (AHCPR 1990).

In addition to sponsoring the development of clinical guidelines, the Medical Treatment Effectiveness Program, or MEDTEP as the AHCPR initiative is named, will examine the effectiveness of various ways to disseminate guidelines and will develop data bases that are useful for patient outcomes research and clinical decision making. The rationale for establishing such an entity and supporting such research is "evidence that health care practitioners will voluntarily change their practice behavior when pertinent information about practice patterns and patient outcomes is available to them," a rationale that likewise underlies the use of clinical guidelines as controls on the volume and intensity of services (AHCPR 1990).

The main problem in developing clinical guidelines is that it is precisely in the areas in which guidelines would be the most useful that we have the least information on which to base them. That is, it is in clinical situations in which information on effectiveness and cost-effectiveness is incomplete, contradictory, or controversial that guidelines would have the greatest impact. In these circumstances, however, prematurely developed guidelines could do substantial harm, even if they do reduce cost, by inhibiting development of further knowledge about a procedure or by forcing conformity before knowledge is precise enough to determine what works (or what could work) and what does not.

## Factors Thought to Influence the Effectiveness of Guidelines

Because there is no enforcement associated with the issuance of guidelines, at least in the scenario considered here, the success of guidelines in changing practice patterns depends in large part on the acceptance of the recommendations by physicians. But guidelines are needed most when there is considerable variation in practice; thus, a given recommendation will always be contrary to the usual practice of a substantial portion of physicians.

How can guidelines be made most persuasive? If there is real "professional uncertainty," as opposed to polarized opinion, about the appropriateness of a particular practice, an authoritative guideline would be expected to have a greater chance of influencing practice. Beyond that, however, the extent to which physicians agree with the objectives of the guideline and approve of the actual development process itself will be important to its persuasiveness. Thus, to maximize acceptance of a guideline's recommendation, the process of development should be open and clearly defined, should allow for direct clinical input, and should be perceived of as objectively assessing the relevant information.

To develop scientifically sound guidelines, input is needed from several sources: physicians who have substantial expertise in the clinical practice being assessed; physicians who have a broad clinical perspective; and experts in the methodologies of assessment, including study design, data analysis, information synthesis, health outcomes, and costs of care. Advice must be obtained not only from the relevant physician subspecialists and primary care physicians, but also from clinical epidemiologists, statisticians, decision analysts, and economists. Further, because the objectives of guidelines are multifaceted, payers, insurers, and beneficiaries should also be involved in guideline development. Predetermined standards of evidence and decision making should be applied.

Ideally, guidelines should be based on objective data. Primary clinical data from well-designed studies are in short supply, however, and thus are rarely available in sufficient quantity to be the sole basis for a guideline. Information on the impact of clinical services on patient function and outcomes is sorely lacking, as are data on patient preferences and utilities among various alternatives. The practical and economic issues involved make it infeasible for individual providers to collect such data. As noted above, the newly formed national Agency for Health Care Policy and Research is an important advancement in this area and promises to make significant contributions to the information and knowledge needed for guideline development.

Methods used to evaluate secondary data (e.g., meta-analysis, decision analysis, and simulation techniques) also are important sources of information for the development of clinical guidelines. However, because both primary and secondary data are typically limited, expert opinion must play an important role. Disagreement and conflict are implicit in any task that involves making decisions under conditions of considerable uncertainty. Methods to resolve such conflicts in the most valid, reliable fashion are not well developed, which often detracts from the guideline's effectiveness in changing practice patterns.

Decisions must also be made regarding whether a particular guideline should be oriented toward a specific technology or service (e.g., appropriate utilization of the exercise stress test) as opposed to the management of a given clinical condition (such as appropriate diagnostic and therapeutic management of patients who are suspected of having coronary artery disease). Generally, most medical practices offer some benefit to selected patients in specific clinical circumstances; few services or procedures are useless. Guidelines, therefore, will need to refer to both of these dimensions, but their orientation will influence their usefulness to various physicians.

## Feasibility of Guideline Development

Because nearly all medical services offer some potential benefit, the utilization issues surrounding medical practice generally concern the marginal net benefits and costs of specific interventions. Although a great deal has been learned about the identification and measurement of these benefits and costs, analysis of the cost-effectiveness of medical practices remains controversial. Much more research concerning the methodology appropriate to the measurement of costs and outcomes is required to develop high-quality, broadly accepted guidelines.

The development of well-crafted, high-quality guidelines that will be well accepted by physicians is expensive. Based on the experience of organizations that have developed or are developing guidelines, the process has been estimated to cost between $10,000 and $500,000 per guideline, depending on the sophistication of the methods used to analyze and synthesize available inputs and then design and modify the criteria. Less elaborate approaches, such as gathering expert opinion or performing a cursory review of published literature, may be much less costly. On the other hand, more extensive projects involving generation of new data on cost or effectiveness may be much more expensive.

In addition to the financial costs of development, the use of guidelines is associated with a variety of nonfinancial costs. These include the risks of prematurely entrenching practice patterns and eliminating the potential for future improvements, reducing or eliminating appropriate variations, such as those that respond to patient-specific factors or preferences, and adding complexity (and antagonism) to what will be more frequent appeals for exceptions to guidelines.

It will probably never be feasible to develop guidelines for many clinical practices, because the range of issues to be addressed would be vast and the cost considerable. Therefore, the scope and effectiveness of whatever guidelines are developed should be maximized. This can be accomplished in at least two ways. First, developing guidelines for new practices offers great potential for shaping patterns of care in appropriate ways, thereby preventing inappropriate use before it becomes widespread. Second, when developing guidelines for existing services, effectiveness can be enhanced by focusing on practices that are provided in great volume, have high aggregate financial costs, present significant risks or benefits, and are susceptible to considerable disagreement regarding appropriate use (as manifested by variations in utilization or significant differences of opinion among experts).

## Effectiveness as a Volume Control

### Empirical evidence

Reports of the effectiveness of clinical guidelines in influencing medical practice have been mixed. To some degree, this is undoubtedly because a variety of types of guidelines and methods of dissemination have been studied. As mentioned earlier, guidelines can be developed for two purposes: to inform, educate, and guide providers (especially physicians), and to control service utilization. These different types of guidelines can then be disseminated in various ways; for example, with or without education, with or without penalties, with or without the support of clinical leaders, and so forth. Review of the literature on the effectiveness of guidelines is complicated by these variations. Moreover, much of the empirical work in this area has been done in the inpatient setting rather than in ambulatory practice, so any application of these results to Medicare's Part B program or to insurance plans that cover outpatient services should be done with care.

Perhaps the most compelling work that supports the use of guidelines comes from Wennberg in collaboration with the Maine Medical Association (Wennberg 1985; PPRC 1988). Early evidence from this project suggests that information as simple as feedback that shows a physician his or her own practice patterns in relation to a small group of peers can be effective in altering patterns that deviate from the statistical norm. In addition to this direct influence on practice, such an approach has been reported to stimulate research on the relationship between various rates of service utilization and outcomes of care (Wennberg 1985).

In his review of the effectiveness of various methods of influencing physician behavior, Eisenberg (1985, 1986) found that such feedback is particularly useful as an adjunct to educational guidelines. The most effective feedback is provided in a personal manner by a respected professional, tailored to the particular physician, and reflective of current or recent practice data. Such feedback can be expensive, however. In their study of physician education coupled with chart audit and feedback, Schroeder et al. (1984) found that the relatively small financial savings produced by giving feedback appeared to be negated by the costs of the program.

The effects of educational guidelines (i.e., those that are based on outcomes research or consensus of expert opinion and that suggest clinically appropriate care) appear to depend substantially on the method of dissemination (Eisenberg 1985). Although most studies suggest that the simple transfer of information is not effective in changing practice, certain factors appear to enhance effectiveness. These include the use of computer reminders, the commitment of clinical leaders, personal as opposed to impersonal transfer of information, and an environment in which physicians are open to change. A study of the effect on physician practice of the recommendations of the Consensus Development Program of the National Institutes of Health supports this conclusion: with results simply published in a leading professional journal, little effect was seen on practice (Kosecoff et al. 1987). Similarly, a survey of the practice patterns of internists demonstrated relatively low levels of compliance with the cancer-screening guidelines of the American Cancer Society and with the immunization guidelines of the Centers for Disease Control (Schwartz et al. 1991).

The most successful use of guidelines seems to occur in conjunction with extensive peer involvement, financial incentives, or both. In a program conducted by the Maine Medical Association, for example, prostatectomy rates declined in the state after urologists received feedback comparing their utilization rates with those of their peers (AMA 1986). This feedback was accompanied by information on the outcomes of the procedure. Because this program was conducted by the Maine Medical Association, it had substantial credibility. Reductions in hysterectomy rates were observed in Saskatchewan using a similar program (Dyck et al. 1977). Broad decreases in the use of ancillary services were observed by a Pennsylvania Blue Shield program that compared providers' utilization rates with those of their peers as part of Pennsylvania Blue Shield's utilization review efforts (Schwartz et al. 1988).

There appears to be some asymmetry in the impact of guidelines, in that recommendations to increase practices may be more readily accepted than those that suggest that practice volumes should decrease. For example, compliance with recommendations to obtain Pap smears, to test stool for occult blood, and to immunize patients against influenza have been better accepted than recommendations to reduce or eliminate the use of chest radiographs for screening (Schwartz et al. 1991). Although this observation suggests that physicians' economic incentives are operative, this is not uniformly the case, particularly when the procedure involves some risk, discomfort, or substantial expense to the patient. Recommendations that sigmoidoscopy be used to screen for the early detection of colon cancer and that mammography be used to screen for the early detection of breast cancer have been less well accepted than simpler, safer, less expensive cancer-screening tests and procedures, even when the physician derives substantial financial gain from the performance of the riskier procedure (Schwartz et al. 1991).

Guidelines that have been developed with the substantial involvement of the affected physicians and that are well accepted by physicians appear to have greater impact than controversial guidelines developed without significant input from physicians. In addition, involving professional societies and their representatives in the development of guidelines is useful and desirable for expediting acceptance among providers. Neither practicing gynecologists nor the American College of Obstetrics and Gynecology were significantly involved in the formulation of the American Cancer Society guidelines on the recommended frequency of

Pap smears. Consequently, there was a general lack of acceptance of the guidelines, and ultimately they had to be revised.

We can conclude from the empirical evidence that guidelines appear to be most effective in changing practice when they are accompanied by feedback about an individual physician's practice compared to his or her peers, or when they suggest a change that patients prefer and doctors find easier to recommend, such as a less painful, less invasive procedure to accomplish the same clinical goal.

### Anticipated impacts of guidelines on volume and intensity: A theoretical analysis

What do behavioral and economic theories suggest about the effectiveness of guidelines? To reiterate, the assumption is that there is some effort to educate physicians about the content of given guidelines but that there is no enforcement such as there would be, for example, if physicians were denied reimbursement for practice that did not comply with guidelines. If physicians are true patient agents (of any of the types discussed in Chapter 3), and if they believe a new recommendation is credible, then the guidelines are likely to be accepted regardless of profitability. The effect on aggregate expenditures will depend on the nature of the recommendation. Assuming it is a volume- or cost-control measure, however, aggregate expenditures will decrease.

Profit maximizers will always adopt a recommendation that increases their profit. Target-income physicians, however, might not adopt the recommendation if they are already hitting their target. It must also be assumed that the doctor would like to reach the target by providing a lower volume of services, probably because use of one of the inputs—his or her own time—is a source of disutility. Thus, if the use of specific recommended services is more profitable than were those used previously, overall volume and costs are likely to increase for both profit-maximizing and income-targeting physicians.

What if the guidelines result in lower profits for the physician, as they likely would if instituted as a control on volume or costs? The profit maximizer will be resistant to the new guidelines unless, over the long term, his or her patients realize that their physician is offering or recommending a nonpreferred service. Should this realization result in a greater decline in demand for the physician's services over the long term than the physician would have experienced because of adopting the guidelines, the physician will eventually adopt the new guidelines. Thus, even guidelines that reduce a physician's short-term profits may be widely adopted, but perhaps only over the long term. It is particularly important to the effectiveness of the guidelines as a volume control in this scenario that the public be well aware of the recommendation or be able to judge the quality of care.

The physician seeking a target income will generally accept a recommendation that lowers profits more readily than a profit-maximizing physician will, because the former balances income with other goals of practice such as the psychic gain of serving the patient's interest. When adhering to the guidelines involves substantial increases in the physician's own time commitment, without an offsetting increase in revenues, resistance may be greater. More generally, informing the doctor that current practice may actually harm patients will increase the disutility cost of demand inducement for that procedure, thereby making physicians less eager to induce demand. Information on the costliness of procedures that do no harm would be expected to have less impact, especially if patients are well insured. The effect of guidelines on aggregate expenditures will depend on whether (and which) other services are increased to maintain income. A guideline will likely improve the quality of care for the condition or service it addresses, but it may have adverse effects on the quality of other care because of the shift in services.

## Summary and Conclusions

Given the extent of what appears to be inappropriate use of health services in the U.S. health care system, an effective program of guideline development, especially if coupled with other effective interventions, can be expected to result in sizable reductions in the volume of services provided and their associated costs. Based on the literature, it is not possible to provide an accurate estimate of the level of savings. However, based on the experiences of those who have been involved in guideline development and use, it seems reasonable to expect a savings of 10 percent in direct and induced costs without any net loss of benefit (and perhaps with some gain in benefit). The savings realized from the development and application of guidelines can be significant and recurring. The application of guidelines to new practices also offers the opportunity to reduce the rate of increase of volume and costs.

In addition to the direct volume- and cost-control benefits derived from the development of guidelines, a number of important external benefits accrue. Guidelines may contribute to a reduction in the practice of defensive medicine by providing physicians with support for the decision not to proceed with a practice that is of doubtful value. Perhaps most importantly, when used in conjunction with other cost-containment efforts, guidelines can help build confidence that these other efforts will not compromise the quality of patient care. Thus, guidelines can serve to strengthen confidence and broaden support for concurrent cost-containment efforts. If physicians fear that malpractice suits will result from not using services, then guidelines could reassure them of the safety of omitting relatively useless tests or treatment.

Guidelines also offer the potential in the intermediate and long term to affect provider decision making. A reorientation toward considering issues of cost and cost-effectiveness trade-offs in clinical decision making should result in more appropriate, cost-effective care in the long term.

Scientifically derived guidelines offer the potential to improve provider information and to improve the quality and cost-effectiveness of medical care. In fact, such programs probably are necessary, at some level, to achieve such changes in practice. However, although necessary, guidelines almost certainly are not sufficient in and of themselves to cause substantial reductions in inappropriate utilization in the short or intermediate term. The most effective interventions appear to depend on multiple components of education, financial incentives, peer values, and administrative changes. The development of guidelines should therefore be perceived as an important component of volume- and cost-control mechanisms. Guidelines should be integrated with efforts to provide financial incentives for cost-effective care (e.g., denial of payment, sharing in savings, and market pressure from patients who share in the cost of care), efforts to reorient providers' perspectives (e.g., professional societies, peer practice comparisons, and public opinion), efforts to include a service's cost-effectiveness as a factor in decision making, and efforts to expand utilization review.

# References

Agency for Health Care Policy and Research (AHCPR), U.S. Department of Health and Human Services. 1990. *AHCPR Program Note*. Rockville, MD: AHCPR.

American Academy of Pediatrics. 1938. *Report of the Committee on Immunization Procedures of the American Academy of Pediatrics*. Evanston, IL: American Academy of Pediatrics.

American Cancer Society. 1988. *Summary of Current Guidelines for the Cancer-Related Checkup*. Atlanta: American Cancer Society.

American Medical Association (AMA), Department of Health Care Review, Division of Health Policy and Program Evaluation. 1986. *Confronting Regional Variations: The Maine Approach*. Chicago: AMA.

American Medical Association (AMA), Office of Quality Assurance. 1989. *Listing of Practice Parameters, Guidelines, and Technology Assessments*. Chicago: AMA.

Centers for Disease Control (CDC), Immunization Practices Advisory Committee, U.S. Department of Health and Human Services. 1989. "General Recommendations on Immunization." *Morbidity and Mortality Weekly* 38: 205–14, 219–27.

Chassin, M. R., et al. 1989. *The Appropriateness of Selected Medical and Surgical Procedures: Relationship to Geographic Variations.* Ann Arbor, MI: Health Administration Press.

Dixon, A. S. 1990. "The Evolution of Clinical Policies." *Medical Care* 28: 201–20.

Dyck, F. J., F. A. Murphy, J. K. Murphy, D. A. Road, M. S. Boyd, E. Osborne, D. DeVlieger, B. Korchinski, C. Ripley, A. T. Bromley, and P. B. Innes. 1977. "Effect of Surveillance on the Number of Hysterectomies in the Province of Saskatchewan." *New England Journal of Medicine* 296: 1326–28.

Eisenberg, J. M. 1985. "Physician Utilization: The State of Research about Physicians' Practice Patterns." *Medical Care* 23: 461–83.

———. 1986. *Doctors' Decisions and the Cost of Medical Care.* Ann Arbor, MI: Health Administration Press.

Fletcher, R. H., and S. W. Fletcher. 1990. "Clinical Practice Guidelines." *Annals of Internal Medicine* 113: 645–46.

Jacoby, I. 1985. "The Consensus Development Program of the National Institutes of Health: Current Practices and Historical Perspectives." *International Journal of Technology Assessment in Health Care* 1: 420–32.

Kosecoff, J., D. E. Kanouse, W. H. Rogers, L. McCloskey, C. M. Winslow, and R. H. Brook. 1987. "Effects of the National Institutes of Health Consensus Development Program on Physician Practice." *Journal of the American Medical Association* 258: 2708–13.

Morris, L. C. 1987. "Introduction to the Blue Cross and Blue Shield Association Guidelines." In *Common Diagnostic Tests: Use and Interpretation,* edited by H. C. Sox, Jr. Philadelphia: American College of Physicians.

Physician Payment Review Commission (PPRC). 1988. *Annual Report to Congress.* Washington, DC: PPRC.

Schroeder, S. A., L. P. Meyers, S. J. McPhee, J. A. Showstack, D. Simborg, S. A. Chapman, and J. K. Leang. 1984. "The Failure of Physician Education as a Cost Containment Strategy. Report of a Prospective Controlled Trial at a University Hospital." *Journal of the American Medical Association* 252: 225–300.

Schwartz, J. S., C. E. Lewis, C. Clancy, M. S. Kinosian, M. H. Radany, and J. P. Koplan. 1991. "Internists' Practices in Health Promotion and Disease Prevention: A Survey." *Annals of Internal Medicine* 114: 46–53.

Schwartz, J. S., S. V. Williams, D. K. Kitz, and J. S. Eisenberg. 1988. "Effectiveness of a Statewide Utilization Review Program Using Profile Analysis." Photocopy.

Wennberg, J. E. 1985. "Commentary on Patient Need, Equity, Supplier-Induced Demand, and the Need to Assess the Outcome of Common Medical Practices." *Medical Care* 23: 512–21.

White, L. J., and J. R. Ball. 1985. "The Clinical Efficacy Assessment Project of the American College of Physicians." *International Journal of Technology Assessment in Health Care* 1: 169–74.

Woolf, S. H. 1990. "Practice Guidelines: A New Reality in Medicine—Recent Developments." *Archives of Internal Medicine* 150: 1811–18.

# Chapter 6

# Utilization Review

Utilization review (UR) was started during World War II when internal hospital committees were created to monitor utilization in an effort to free up beds (Payne 1987). At its inception, UR was concurrent peer review of inpatient care by the physicians on a hospital's staff. Since those early days, many different UR techniques have been developed. Today, according to Ermann (1988), utilization review, is "the collection of techniques in which a third party (other than the patient and the patient's physician) determines the appropriateness of medical services suggested to or provided to the patient by the attending physician." The third party may be the payer, an agent of the payer (such as a vendor of UR services), or a provider (such as a hospital or an HMO).

Utilization review methods have an important common problem: they all need to specify criteria that determine appropriate and inappropriate (or approved and unapproved) services and procedures. Most UR methods currently in use apply to inpatient hospital care and are generally applied to the process of care, not to its outcome or efficacy (Payne 1987). The purpose of UR and the methods used to enforce it vary across organizations and over time. Results can be used to do the following things:

1. Provide feedback to providers; for example, a comparison of a physician's practice patterns with those of a similar group of other physicians

2. Assist in the education of providers, often in combination with practice guidelines or protocols

3. Restrict money benefits available to patients; for example, by imposing financial penalties on patients undertaking surgery without a required second opinion

4. Impose penalties on physicians; for example, by withholding reimbursement and not permitting balance billing

5. Impose penalties on hospitals or other providers; for example, by refusing to pay for admissions or days of stay classified as inappropriate

In this chapter we examine the effectiveness of UR in influencing the volume and intensity of physician services, focusing primarily on UR methods instituted by some agent other than the direct provider of care. UR for internal management purposes will not be of primary concern. Physicians today provide a substantial share of total services (and of the most rapidly growing services) in outpatient settings, including their offices and other nonhospital sites. However, because of the relative lack of literature on the impact of outpatient UR for physician services, inferences must be drawn from studies of UR applied in inpatient settings. Those inferences are made in this chapter, and theoretical analysis is used to predict the potential impact of UR in settings that have not yet been studied or where UR has not been used extensively. Finally, the probable effects of more extensive implementation of UR on Medicare and non-Medicare physician volume are explored.

It is important to begin by looking at the form and apparent impact of the UR methods in each of the six cells in Table 6.1. Methods of UR may be classified along two different dimensions: the time of the review relative to the time of service, and the location of the care. Reviews can be performed before, during, or after the service is provided and may be applied to services provided to inpatients or to outpatients (Ermann 1988). Table 6.1 shows the types of review offered in each setting at each time.

**Table 6.1**   Utilization Review Methods

| Location of Service | Time of Service | | |
|---|---|---|---|
| | *Before* | *During* | *After* |
| Inpatient | Preadmission certification | Concurrent review | Retrospective discharge or claims review |
| | Second surgical opinion | Case management | |
| Outpatient | Preprocedure or precertification review | Concurrent review (episode of treatment review) | Retrospective discharge or claims review |

# Prospective Utilization Review

Prospective UR, which takes place before a service is provided, includes preadmission review, second surgical opinion programs, and precertification or preprocedure review. High-cost case management, or utilization management, is a method that can be used either before or during treatment, but it is discussed in this chapter in the context of concurrent review. Each of the three types of prospective utilization review is outlined below.

### Preadmission review

General preadmission review procedures are intended to affect inpatient admissions by assessing the appropriateness of a decision to admit a patient before the admission takes place. This method usually does not include a determination of whether the diagnostic or therapeutic procedure provided in connection with the admission is itself medically necessary. Rather, preadmission review is generally confined to evaluating the location and timing of the admission (Institute of Medicine 1989).

The use of preadmission procedures varies across programs and organizations. Despite this variability, the following features are common to all programs:

1. Patient- or physician-initiated contact with the review organization as notification of an intention to admit

2. Initial screening of the proposed admission, usually by a nurse reviewer, that will result in approval if the case conforms with established criteria

3. Physician review of cases that do not conform with the criteria

4. An appeals process for proposed admissions judged to be inappropriate

It is clear that the standards or the criteria themselves play an important role in the operation and effectiveness of preadmission review. Restrictive standards may harm patients, cause a great deal of wasted time and delay, and prompt physicians to object to both the administrative work and the final decision. Lenient standards waste resources and ultimately may have no effect because many of the cases reviewed are approved. Precisely where a set of standards lies on a spectrum between "harm or hassle" and "ineffectiveness" is a critical choice for any program.

A variety of such standards exist, and most of them were developed originally for retrospective review in the professional standards review organization (PSRO) program for Medicare or for research on unnecessary hospital use (Payne 1987). The two most commonly used sets of criteria were derived from the Appropriateness Evaluation Protocol (AEP) or from the ISD-A criteria (i.e., intensity of services, severity of illness, discharge, and appropriateness screens). These tools have been adapted for prospective use (Restuccia 1982). The AEP criteria, in the public domain, have been validated and are considered reliable (Restuccia 1982). The ISD-A criteria are private and their validity and reliability have not been established. In addition to these two mechanisms, more explicit medical necessity criteria, developed by Value Health Sciences, are increasingly being used.

Another important factor that influences the effectiveness of and overall satisfaction with preadmission UR is the nature of the communication between physicians and reviewers. Physicians need to use terminology in the initial proposal for admission that matches that used by the review organization. The participation of physician advisers who review the initial denials is key. The physician reviewers are not usually bound by specific predetermined guidelines, but instead they use their experience and judgment to make a determination. In principle, discussions between the attending and advising physicians create an opportunity for the exchange of additional information that can lead to better understanding and agreement regarding proper treatment. However, not all UR plans encourage such communication.

The appeals process varies across organizations. Peer review organizations (PROs) have a formal appeals process that is required by Medicare. In most private organizations the appeals are reviewed by a physician, medical director, or committee of physicians other than those who reviewed the case initially.

The results of denials also can differ. Medicare prohibits hospitals from billing patients for admissions for which Medicare reimbursement is denied. Private insurers, on the other hand, may not be able to prevent hospitals from billing patients when claims are denied.

### Effectiveness of preadmission review

The techniques used to evaluate the effectiveness of preadmission review vary from simple before-and-after comparisons to quasi-experimental designs or analyses using multivariate regression models. The most common technique is to study changes in use that occur following a program's implementation. For example, Kauer (1983) reported that inpatient days fell 21 percent over a three-year period following the start of a preadmission program, suggesting an 11 to 1 benefit-to-cost ratio. Cure, a preadmission UR program established in Northeastern Ohio by

Blue Cross, reported a 13 percent drop in inpatient days in the first five months and claimed an estimated $30 million in savings (Shahoda 1984). Both programs were introduced in the mid-1980s, when inpatient days for Medicare and non-Medicare patients were dropping nationwide. It is not clear, therefore, how much of the cost reduction is attributable to the UR program rather than to the nation's overall drop in inpatient days.

Preauthorization programs, as judged by before-and-after studies, appear to be effective in Medicaid settings and in preferred provider organizations (PPOs). A California Medicaid preauthorization program claimed a 5.5 to 1 benefit-to-cost ratio (Wickizer 1990). A California PPO reported a 20 percent decrease in inpatient costs, although the program's introduction also was associated with a 152 percent increase in ambulatory surgery (Holahan and Stuart 1977). Similarly, a Florida PPO that provides coverage to Dade County Public School employees found that inpatient days decreased (by 11.5 percent) but that outpatient surgery increased (by 47.1 percent) (Graugnard 1987).

These simple studies do not control for the effects of other influences that may be occurring at the same time. Comparative studies, in which the experience in the area where the program was introduced is compared to another (ideally similar) place that had no program change, are somewhat better than simple studies. Comparative studies, however, rely heavily on the assumption that all other influences affect the two sites in the same way and to the same extent. A 1985 RCA Company study revealed a substantially larger decline in inpatient utilization for employees in plants that had prior utilization review compared to plants that did not use the program (O'Donnell 1987). Surgical days increased for both groups, but to a larger extent for the unmanaged group. Because other days declined, however, the overall effect was a 4 percent drop in benefit costs in the places that had prior review, compared to a 6 percent increase in the unmanaged group. The Service Employees International Union measured the impact of precertification against a control group and against an estimate of the expected results had the program not been initiated. When measured against expected results over a two-year period, the precertification program registered a greater decline in inpatient days, whereas when measured against the statewide control group, inpatient days under the precertification plan declined the first year but not the second.

Multivariate analyses present a more mixed picture of the effect of prior review. Using quarterly claims data, Scheffler, Gibbs, and Gurnick (1987) studied the impact of preadmission review for Blue Cross patients. They used multivariate regression to control for the effect of prospective payment and other Blue Cross cost-management efforts. They found that preadmission review was associated with lower hospital admissions and lower outpatient visit rates, but that it did not affect hospital or outpatient expenditures. Lower rates were offset by higher unit costs. In partial contrast, Zuckerman (1987) found that states with prior authorization programs did experience lower growth in Medicaid expenditures over the period 1977–1984, other things being equal.

Overall, preauthorization programs appear to substantially affect inpatient use initially, but their impact on total spending is not as great, and rates of change in both use and cost eventually return to levels achieved without intervention.

## Second surgical opinion programs

As prior authorization programs specifically focused on elective surgery, second surgical opinion programs differ from more generic programs in two ways: the insured receives a second opinion service (either voluntarily or under threat of lower benefits or other sanctions), and typically no penalty results from undertaking a surgical procedure even after a negative second opinion.

A patient who wishes to receive a surgical procedure is required to consult two physicians. A positive recommendation or agreement from the first physician is followed by a review of that opinion by a second physician; the review addresses the necessity and location (inpatient or outpatient) of the proposed surgery. Most second surgical opinion programs usually are concerned with 15 to 30 common discretionary surgical procedures. The trend over time is for programs to target smaller numbers of procedures for second opinions. Procedures for which a second opinion is almost never adverse are dropped. Some programs are voluntary: they simply represent a willingness of the insurer to cover the cost of a second opinion and to assist in arranging for that opinion. Others are mandatory in the sense that if there is no second opinion, the insurer or employer reduces its payment for the surgery by some percentage, and the patient must make up the difference in cost. The covered charges subject to the penalty may include physician fees and, in some cases, facility charges.

In 1989, 53 percent of the nation's conventional health insurance plans and 62 percent of managed care plans offered mandatory second surgical opinion programs (HIAA 1990, p. 33; Sullivan and Rice 1991). According to a recent Wyatt Company survey of 800 medium and large U.S. companies, 48 percent of employers have mandatory second opinion programs and 45 percent have voluntary programs (Wyatt Company 1991). Twelve states require second surgical opinions for Medicaid recipients (HCFA 1991, pp. 71, 74).

Either the patient or the first surgeon is responsible for arranging for the second opinion. Insurers usually assemble a panel of surgeons and surgical specialists to provide the opinions. The reviewers cannot accept the patient as their own and cannot review patients of surgeons with whom they have close contact (Rutgow and Sieverts 1989). The insurer will usually pay for the surgery regardless of the second surgeon's opinion. In a small subset of mandatory second opinion programs, benefits are reduced or denied if the second opinion is negative, unless a third opinion overrules the second.

### Effectiveness of second surgical opinion programs

The literature on second opinion surgery has been reviewed extensively by Rutgow and Sieverts (1989) and by Lindsey and Newhouse (1990). None of the studies these authors reviewed had a proper control group design that provided reliable estimates of the impact of second opinion surgery on surgical rates and expenditures. Despite the absence of valid studies, the general consensus is that voluntary second opinion surgery programs do not affect the rate of surgeries and do not result in cost savings (Parks 1983). The empirical evidence concerning the effect of mandatory second opinion surgery is thought to suggest some impact on surgery rates and expenditures.

In a 1974 study, McCarthy and Widmer (1974) evaluated the impact of second opinion surgery for inpatient and outpatient services. Two groups were evaluated. The first group comprised 20,000 self-insured union members for whom a second opinion program was mandatory but not strictly enforced. Of this group, 602 patients recommended for surgery submitted to second opinion, and 17.6 percent of those did not receive a confirming second opinion. In the second group (200,000 patients), a second opinion was entirely voluntary. For this second, voluntary group, a total of 754 patient records were available, with a 30.4 percent nonconfirmation rate. The authors estimated that the overall program achieved an 8 to 1 benefit-cost ratio. Ruchlin, Finkel, and McCarthy (1982) also estimated a positive benefit-cost ratio for a mandatory second opinion program applied to inpatient and outpatient surgeries, but at a much lower ratio of 2.6 to 1. Tyson (1985) reported a similar benefit-to-cost ratio (2.63 to 1) in evaluating the Cornell–New York Hospital's mandatory second opinion program. After six months, more than eight out of every ten nonconfirmed patients still had not had surgery. Other programs have reported similar results (National Health Policy Forum 1986; Business Insurance 1985).

Medicaid is the program closest to Medicare from an administrative point of view, although the two programs treat different populations. Medicaid has 13 mandatory second opinion programs (Lindsey 1989). Poggio et al. (1985) evaluated the Massachusetts Medicaid Program and attributed a 1.9 percent reduction in the rate of surgery to mandatory second opinion programs.

Second opinion surgery programs can be measured in terms of their direct impact and their secondary effect. The former, which is the impact on patients whose surgical needs are being assessed, has been found to be relatively small, resulting in about a 10 percent reduction in surgery rates for the cases considered (Poggio et al. 1985). The secondary effect is also referred to as the sentinel effect because physicians, knowing that their recommendations are reviewed, may choose to change their behavior. The sentinel effect has been estimated to account for 90 percent of the reduction in second opinion surgeries. Lindsey and Newhouse (1990) note, however, that because this effect has not been measured against true control groups, it must be treated with caution. Furthermore, the health consequences of the sentinel effect are not known.

In summary, studies of second opinion surgery have not produced consistent empirical evidence that this technique is effective in changing utilization patterns. Whereas early studies have claimed significant impact, later studies have not reinforced this conclusion. All studies may be affected by methodological problems. Moreover, as the scope of surgical procedures subject to second opinion has been narrowed over time, even a moderately high benefit-to-cost ratio has not translated into substantial total savings. According to the Institute of Medicine (1989), most private UR companies currently do not view second opinion surgery as an effective cost-containment procedure. Research does suggest that second opinion programs might have a sentinel effect that could be substantial, but such an effect is not a strong motivation for any single insurer, especially one with a modest market share.

The effects of second surgical opinion on quality of care are less certain. There is no clear evidence that unconfirmed surgeries are medically unnecessary. Without a study of the long-term impact of delayed surgery and without comparisons to appropriate control groups, there is no reason to believe that the surgeries not performed should necessarily be eliminated. The data show savings, but the costs of alternative medical care services usually are not counted, and the costs to patients are not included in the analyses. Although in the short run the use of surgery might be reduced, in the long run the costs of alternative medical treatment, including possible delayed surgery, are not necessarily reduced.

## Precertification review for outpatient services

The components of precertification or preprocedure review for outpatient services are similar to those for inpatient admissions or surgery. The patient or attending physician must contact the review organization and report the intended procedure. Outpatient UR is usually much more selective than preadmission screening. Only certain high-cost outpatient procedures, such as magnetic resonance imaging, are subject to the requirement. Moreover, outpatient UR does not consider the location of the procedure, but assumes that the outpatient setting is always cheaper if the procedure is to be performed at all. What *is* questioned is the need for and timing of the service.

Outpatient UR is less well developed than inpatient screening, so it should not be surprising that there are few studies of its effects. The lack of multivariate or valid comparative studies limits us to considering before-and-after studies and anecdotal information. Intracorp, a UR firm, reports that its preclaims appropriateness review could produce a net saving (Leland 1990). Zalta (1990) argues, however, that the number of review requests is likely to be high and the number of denials relatively low. He conjectures, for example, that a program to screen requests for electrocardiograms might reject as many as half of them, but that the costs of operating the program would be more than twice the savings from reduced tests.

## Effectiveness of precertification review

As noted earlier, *inpatient* preadmission review is already prevalent. Although it seems to generate modest savings, whatever effects it might have on physician services have occurred already in plans that have a UR program in place. Thus, the relevant question for both Medicare and for private insurers is whether extending pretreatment approval programs (e.g., to outpatient settings) is likely to generate greater savings. Based on the limited empirical evidence, there is not much reason to be optimistic. Even when applied to high-cost procedures, precertification or preprocedure review appears to generate only small savings. It is difficult to believe that the direct savings could be larger when the review is applied to services currently not covered, especially outpatient physician services. There might be a larger sentinel effect, but the direct effects of such programs are unlikely to be large enough to justify their cost.

If it were possible to routinize and codify a set of indications for selected high-volume outpatient procedures, and if requests could be computerized and processed cheaply, outpatient precertification might be able to pay its own way. The technology to implement such a system has yet to be developed, however. The alternative is to strengthen inpatient preadmission screening; Medicare, in particular, now has a relatively weak screening program. Even mandatory second surgical opinion programs, the strongest of the lot, show only modest savings.

To save more money, programs would have to reject many more admissions than they do now—and that could generate adverse effects on quality.

## Concurrent Utilization Review

There are few pure concurrent review programs. The objective of concurrent review is to alter the pattern of services to be rendered in the future. It is intrinsically a kind of prior approval mechanism, although it is put in place after care has been initiated for an illness. Moreover, most of the empirical analyses report on programs that combine formal preadmission review with concurrent review. Accordingly, this section covers both concurrent review programs and programs that combine pretreatment and concurrent review.

### Case management

The primary form of concurrent review is case management, which is usually (although not always) limited to episodes of illness expected to result in high costs. The insured person is encouraged or required to contact a case manager, who can authorize coverage of services not typically covered by the insurance contract. Case management is "a set of techniques intended to promote more cost-effective and appropriate modes of care for patients with expensive illnesses" (Institute of Medicine 1989). *Cost-effective* here must mean *lower cost*, because case management techniques do not use methods to determine the value of different outcomes in order to compare them with the cost of different patient treatment processes. This approach is most common among conventional insurers, although cost-management services also are offered to self-insured plans (Henderson and Wallack 1987).

Case management is usually different from (but often coordinated with) the medical management of the patient's illness. Patient needs and circumstances are assessed and needed services are then planned, facilitated, and monitored (Institute of Medicine 1989). Cost savings are expected to result from the program's ability to coordinate services and to substitute lower-cost services for higher-cost services.

There is no evidence on the frequency with which patients decline the opportunity for case management. Some patients do see case management as bothersome, and physicians also are thought to have mixed reactions. They may be unaware of all the services available, unfamiliar with their patients' insurance benefits, and reluctant to go to the trouble of discussing treatment with the case manager. Being informed of possible additional insurance benefits to patients tends to cause physicians to cooperate more with the program (Institute of Medicine 1989).

## *Effectiveness of case management*

This technique has not been subject to rigorous review as a stand-alone program. Case management firms sometimes generate estimates of savings by first asking case managers to estimate what the cost of the patient's treatment episode would have been had there been no intervention, and then comparing that estimate with the actual cost. Somewhat more valid studies try to compare case-managed patients with other supposedly similar patients. However, due to self-selection bias and the absence of a true control group, we have little evidence on actual effectiveness.

The other relevant issue in estimating total program savings is the relative number of high-cost patients suitable for case management. Although it is true that health insurance, like all insurance, tends to pay large benefits to a small number of insured persons, not all high-cost illnesses are suitable for case management. The technique is more suited to chronic illness or illnesses that cover a long time span than to short-term acute illnesses.

## Concurrent and pretreatment review combined

In a recent series of studies, data from one private insurance company were used to evaluate the cumulative impact of preadmission certification and concurrent review on utilization (Feldstein, Wickizer, and Wheeler 1988; Wickizer, Wheeler, and Feldstein 1989; Wickizer 1990). Using multivariate regression analysis and controlling for many covariates, the researchers compared companies that used the two techniques against companies that did not. The work this group of researchers performed is the best analysis to date, although the results reflect the experience of only one insurer and the groups were not randomly sampled.

Feldstein, Wickizer, and Wheeler (1988) evaluated the impact of UR programs in which participation was mandatory and penalties were imposed on patients. The researchers used a combination of cross-sectional and longitudinal analyses (evaluating two years of program activity) that included controls for differences in case mix, employee characteristics, market factors, and benefit plan features. Three UR methods were used: preadmission certification, concurrent review, and on-site utilization review. The UR program resulted in a 12.3 percent reduction in hospital admissions, an 11.9 percent reduction in total hospital inpatient expenditures, and an 8.3 percent reduction in total medical expenditures per insured person. The researchers concluded that the review program resulted in a one-time reduction in use and costs but had little impact on their growth over time. The researchers also compared groups that had high utilization prior to review to groups that had low prior utilization. The former were found to have significant decreases in use and costs, which was not true among the latter. The benefit-cost ratios were 8.7 to 1 for all groups with UR and 28.3 to 1 for groups with high prior utilization.

When Wickizer, Wheeler, and Feldstein (1989) analyzed three years of data in a follow-up study, the results did not change significantly. Utilization review reduced admissions by 13.1 percent, total inpatient expenditures by 10.7 percent, and total medical expenditures by 5.9 percent. These changes represented reductions in the level of utilization and expenditures, but UR did not affect the rates of change over time (i.e., the growth rates) in these areas (Wickizer 1990). Although the groups compared in this study were not randomly selected, selectivity tests did not show a bias.

Aetna Life Insurance Company reported similar results from the impact of its utilization management program (Allen and Khandker 1988). The study (also combining concurrent and pretreatment review) controlled for some claimant groups, as well as benefit plan differences across the two nonrandom samples of persons subject to review and not subject to review. The multivariate analysis also included a time-trend variable. Hospital admission rates dropped nearly 8 percent for the program sample but only 1 percent for the nonprogram sample. In-hospital days per 1,000 covered persons dropped about 4 percent for the program population and 2 percent for the control group. Surgical outpatient costs per employee increased at about the same rate for both groups (15.5 percent and 16.1 percent, respectively), but inpatient medical and surgical costs rose less rapidly for the UR program sample than for the nonprogram sample. Gross savings from utilization management were estimated at about 12 percent during the period.

Prospective and concurrent inpatient UR appears to have some effect on private-sector inpatient admissions, although not on lengths of stay. The extent of the impact appears to depend on the type of services provided and on initial conditions. The impact of the program also appears to depend on the quality of the review program itself, the reliability of its standards, and the quality of the communication between the attending physician and the utilization reviewers. A successful preadmission program, however, increases the volume and intensity of outpatient services. The inability to reduce lengths of stay indicates that it is harder to affect physicians' decisions regarding the actual treatment than it is to change the location of treatment.

## Retrospective Utilization Review

Retrospective UR is based on hospital discharge or claims records. The most common form compares a provider's aggregate utilization profile to a set standard. Other forms investigate the process of care, as described in discharge or chart records, with the cases for review selected on the basis of high cost, outlier lengths of stay, or even at random. Both the provider profile approach and the medical evaluation strategy are discussed in this chapter. The sanctions that are imposed if review is negative vary, from denial of payment through denial of some or all reimbursement to identification of expensive users.

Large-scale use of retrospective UR began in 1972 with the establishment of professional standards review organizations in the Medicare program. The PSROs analyzed data that profiled utilization patterns as well as data from medical utilization studies. Their major goal was to ensure that utilization of the Part A benefit, either admission rates or length of stay, was not excessive. Medicare replaced the PSRO program in 1983 with the prospective payment system and with a new UR structure, the peer review organization (PRO). The prospective payment system provided strong internal incentives to hospitals to reduce lengths of stay, possibly by the use of a hospital's own UR program. Unlike PSROs, the PROs were intended to ensure that lengths of stay were not too short, although they continued to monitor excessive admissions as well (with the objective of reviewing 25 percent of Medicare admissions).

Since 1986, PROs also have been charged with reviewing other services, especially hospital outpatient departments, health maintenance organizations (HMOs), and competitive medical plans. The PROs are required as well to review hospital readmissions and beneficiary complaints about quality, and to attempt to reduce unnecessary surgery, complications, and avoidable deaths.

Private-sector retrospective UR takes much the same form of comparing provider performance with preset profiles. One important difference between Medicare and private insurance is that Medicare can forbid the hospital to bill the patient for any services that are denied after review, whereas most private insurers do not have the market power to enforce such a ban on extra billing. Moreover, private insurers have a more difficult time than Medicare in extracting refunds of payments judged retrospectively to be inappropriate. Blue Cross plans that have large market shares can copy some of the features of Medicare's plan, as can HMOs, with direct contractual relations with providers.

There has been some discussion of the application of similar methods to outpatient services, and in the case of the PROs and certain ambulatory surgical procedures, some of these methods have actually been implemented. Zalta (1990) considers the profile comparison approach effective in identifying providers who tend to overuse or unbundle, and he advocates using such information in a program to educate physicians. An HMO can drop such individuals from their panels.

## Effectiveness of retrospective UR

The PRO utilization review is usually conducted by a hospital's staff. In addition to retrospective review, the staff must perform concurrent review because it is required to scan admissions within 24 hours of hospitalization. Research has looked at the impact of PSROs as a whole, not at individual components. In the late 1970s, studies came to generally negative conclusions about the impact of PSROs on hospital bed days and costs, although the process of care and the allocation of beds did seem to improve somewhat (Christofferson et al. 1983; Congressional Budget Office 1979). Reviewing this literature, Wickizer (1990) noted that findings of positive effects from PSROs tended to be limited to simple univariate analyses, which did not control for the full spectrum of influences on hospital use and cost.

In studies using Medicare patients as a control group, the government compared the hospital utilization rates of enrollees residing in 18 active PSRO areas and 26 nonactive areas (HCFA 1979). Control and treatment groups were matched and multivariate methods were used. No significant effects on length of stay were discovered. A later study found that PSROs were associated with a 1.58 percent reduction in total days but had no effect on length of stay, which implies that any PSRO effects are limited to effects on admissions (HCFA 1980). The net effect on cost (after adjusting for the cost of administering the program) is therefore small, if it exists at all.

The performance of PROs has yet to undergo a formal analysis. According to Sloan, Morrisey, and Valvona (1988), during the first two years of PRO operation, the average PRO reviewed 45 percent of admissions and denied payment for 2.5 percent of cases. The authors concluded that the PROs were effective in reducing Medicare inpatient admissions, and that some cost savings could be expected.

The literature on the effectiveness of retrospective UR outside the Medicare setting is scant. Buck and White (1974) found a statistically significant reduction in payments for physicians' services in the Medi-Cal program. Medical review committees, which are used to adjudicate payments, did adjust 1 percent of total claims. Brook, Williams, and Ralph (1978) evaluated a program of UR applied to Medicaid claims in New Mexico and found a statistically significant but quite small effect on total claims, at about 0.4 percent of the amount billed. Paris, Salsberg, and Berenson (1979) reviewed a New York Medicaid program targeted at physicians who were high utilizers, and they found a modest direct reduction in expenditures.

## What Do the Empirical Data Show?

The prevailing message from studies of all types of utilization review is that UR can return more than its cost without adversely affecting quality or outcomes. The total savings appear to be small, however. They also appear to be one-time savings rather than a permanent reduction in the rate of growth. This latter conclusion is somewhat surprising, because UR should be able to catch the excessive use of new technologies that drives health care cost growth. Within the set of UR methods, high-cost case management and some types of preadmission screening appear to be most promising.

For the Medicare program and for private insurance programs that already have UR programs in place, there is little evidence that further reductions in volume are feasible with current techniques. Some applications to high-cost outpatient procedures may be possible.

## Conceptual Analysis: Effects of UR on the Volume of Physician Services

The empirical record does not offer much help in analyzing outpatient UR or stronger inpatient UR. We must turn, therefore, to some conceptual considerations: the effectiveness of broader, more intense UR and the consequences of UR-induced volume adjustments on other payers. The physician behavior models discussed in Chapter 3 will prove helpful for the latter task.

There is little doubt that a stronger version of inpatient UR could reduce costs and the volume of inpatient physician services. Any program that denies payment for services that are or might be rendered must eventually reduce the volume of such services and the payments for them. Only in an extreme version of the agency model would physicians continue to render services for which they expect to be paid nothing;

the cost of the complementary hospital inputs would also need to be covered. The stronger the UR program, however, the likelier that there will be some adverse effects on the quality of care. Even concurrent programs reduce quality by subjecting the patient to additional paperwork and delay. This can be seen most clearly in the case of second opinion programs, which require that patients go through the trouble of getting a second opinion. There appear thus far to be minimal health effects. Even if some such effects do occur, they may be small relative to the cost savings, but they will raise the question of a trade-off between cost savings and either hassle or the risk (however slight) of an adverse effect on health.

The real questions, then, about the effectiveness of UR for controlling or limiting the volume of physician services are these: How much quality or well-being, if any, needs to be given up if volumes are to be reduced compared to what they would otherwise have been? Of all the physician services currently rendered, and of all those added to the volume of services each year, how many are useless or harmful, how many have positive benefits that are of less value than their cost, and how many have benefits great enough to justify their cost? Some analysts believe that as many as one-third of all services may fall in the useless or harmful category (no guesses have been made about the proportion of increased or new services in this category). Others set the proportion much lower and argue that substantial cuts in volume or cost require a reduction in the positive benefits that are of less value than their cost. No one has offered a good way of implementing a program to reduce services of this type. After all, how do you judge when services are good but not good enough? Nor has anyone proved that they have a system to capture all of the useless or harmful services. Some "appropriateness" systems do claim to be able to identify some inappropriate services, but the ability to eliminate those services lags behind the ability to identify them—and even that ability is far from a sure thing.

Given the current state of knowledge, it seems fair to conclude that one could make a one-time reduction in inpatient cost (and presumably, volume of physician services) of 5 to 10 percent without producing palpably unacceptable reductions in medical quality. However, these savings in expenditures come at the cost (unknown in size) of extra hassle for patients and physicians. Greater use of these mechanisms in the inpatient setting seems unlikely given the limited current knowledge of which medical services are effective in various circumstances. It is possible that these UR interventions would have more effect if they were combined with other interventions, such as volume targets or relative price changes. If surgery is thought to be overpriced as well as excessive, for example, then cutting the price and adding UR might produce an effect greater than either technique in isolation—and the presence of UR might even guard against underservice (by some standard). In all these cases, experimentation and evaluation seem the best strategies at present.

In the outpatient setting, one can always hope for the invention of an effective system. Realism suggests, however, that any practical system is likely to be less effective than the 5 to 10 percent cost reduction for inpatients. Unless there is some major breakthrough, it seems unlikely that outpatient UR will be a major contributor to reducing outpatient volumes. This is not to deny, however, that the UR may return substantially more than its cost, and therefore be worth doing in special circumstances. Those circumstances may just not be common enough to reduce volumes overall.

Finally, we still await the appearance of a system that can address the *added* services that are the source of the problem of volume growth. Perhaps such new or additional services do not require a special "first difference" UR (although such an approach might make sense in a retrospective review); they may be handled by effective overall UR programs.

The other approach to this issue is to add knowledge about which services are in the useless or modestly useful categories. The current effectiveness initiative of the federal government is pointed in that direction. Some guidelines will surely be developed, and our comments on them would parallel those on past guidelines (as presented in Chapter 5). Utilization review adds fiscal teeth to guidelines, and there is much less on which to base analysis here. Watchful waiting and an open-eyed evaluation would seem to be the best policies for both public and private payers.

## Behavioral Models and Utilization Review

What insights do the behavioral models provide in generating theoretical answers to these empirically unanswered questions? Two issues must be explored: how effective are UR systems likely to be when they are implemented by a single payer, and what effects will they have on other insured persons and other services?

Recall that the profit-maximizing physician induces demand to the maximum, subject to the constraints of competition. A direct and obvious implication is that if one thinks that doctors tend to be profit maximizers and that competition is likely to be a weak check on their behavior, then one would conclude that there should be large volumes of useless, harmful, or low-value services that any UR program of moderate effectiveness could cut. Perhaps the modest impacts of UR so far provide something of a test of this model, but those who take this view should expect UR to be highly effective in controlling volume and of little risk to overall patient well-being.

The agency model is the other model with a simple, but opposite, message. In all versions of this model, the doctor should not be rendering services he or she believes to be harmful. Of course, imperfect information may lead to incorrect beliefs, and UR could be thought of as a way of dealing with physician misinformation by preventing physicians from doing what is harmful, without going to the expense of explaining why. The observation of variations in volumes of physician services across geography is consistent with such an imperfect information approach. What is unknown is whether UR is able to apply better information, whether imperfect information more often leads to lower or higher volume than would be consistent with good information, and whether it really is cheaper, at the margin, to control volume by denying payment than by informing physicians. (Probably both strategies are needed; the question is which one should be pushed further than it is currently.)

A person who believes in the agency model would not expect UR to have much of an effect if that person does not think there is widespread ignorance among physicians about the effectiveness or risk of the services they provide. It does not help much to review the decisions of smart, good doctors. In contrast, the person who believes that doctors are well-intentioned but poorly informed, *and* who imagines that doctors will realize their ignorance and accept UR as a substitute for knowledge, might be more optimistic.

For services of unequivocally positive but small benefit, the agency model is less precise in its implications. The expected behavior depends on which of the agency models one selects. If it is the social agent model, in which the physician is assumed to take account of the cost of services to the population in general as well as the benefits to the individual patient, UR should have either no effect or an adverse one. The reason is that, even in the absence of UR, physicians in this model choose services with consideration for a proper trade-off between costs and benefits, exactly the objective of ideal utilization review. Practical UR may overshoot this objective and still cut volume, but it will do so to excess. In contrast, if the physician behaves as the agent of the individual patient only, he or she will have been providing services of positive but small benefit to insured patients. Utilization review would then be expected to cut volume by the amount of services whose benefits fall short of their costs. Any quantitative sense of how large a cut this would mean requires conjecture about the volume of such clinically beneficial but not cost-beneficial services.

The target-income physician who creates some demand but not the maximum amount would find some of the services he or she recommends disapproved by utilization review. The cut would not be as large as in the profit maximization case, but there would be some cut. The target-income physician might be expected to respond to the consequent reduction in income from the disapproved services by increasing the amount of inducement for other services. (The profit-maximizing physician could not do this because he or she already would have undertaken the maximum amount of inducement for all services.) Although UR also would be used to try to constrain the "bulging balloon" part of total expenses, it would be unlikely to be fully effective. Paradoxically, UR would be expected to be more effective in the case of single-minded profit-maximizing physicians than in the case of target-income physicians.

What effect would successful utilization review implemented by one payer have on volumes of other payers? There are two offsetting influences. On the one hand, some evidence (although it is not conclusive) suggests that UR has a spillover effect on other services for similar conditions rendered to all insured persons. If Medicare were able to use UR to reduce the surgery rate for persons over age 65, then the rate might be expected to fall somewhat for those under age 65 (especially those close in age). This effect would hold for all models of physician behavior except the perfect (patient) agent. On the other hand, in the target-income model, cuts in volume that cut income might cause more demand inducement to persons covered by other insurers. For the same reasons as discussed in the previous paragraph, this behavior would not be expected to occur for profit-maximizing physicians. It does suggest that a strategy of defensive utilization review might be chosen by other insurers.

## Summary and Conclusions

Utilization review is a technique for volume limitation that has enormous conceptual appeal but enormous practical difficulties in implementation. Who could object to perfect UR, which correctly refused to pay for all services whose benefits were less than their cost? On the other hand, who could expect that such perfect UR would ever be practical? Guesses about practical UR depend in large part on prior suspicions about how much volume and how many volume increases are "unnecessary."

Despite years of experience with this technique and substantial interest in it, UR remains surprisingly unevaluated. The normative conclusion about quality is weak because there is no precise way to define necessary and appropriate care. The overall picture of UR's effect on volume is that the techniques developed and accepted for use to date have had modest effects on the level of volume and no effects on the rate of growth in volume. These techniques are likely to have even lesser effects if extended to ambulatory physician services. Breakthroughs may happen, especially with all of the resources currently being devoted to effectiveness research, but until we see the results of that research, UR is unlikely to be a mainstay in attempts to control volume, either for Medicare or for private insurers. It should probably always be incorporated with other techniques, as much for reassurance as for anything else, but the verdict on the overall usefulness of utilization review has still to be delivered.

# References

Allen, H., and R. Khandker. 1988. "Aetna's Health Line Program: Fourth Quarter, 1987 Update." Photocopy.

Brook, R. H., K. N. Williams, and J. E. Ralph. 1978. "Controlling the Use and Cost of Medical Services: The New Mexico Experimental Medical Care Review Organization. A Four Year Case Study." *Medical Care* 10(9): 1–46.

Buck, C. R., Jr., and K. L. White. 1974. "Peer Review: Impact of a System Based on Billing Claims." *New England Journal of Medicine* 291: 877–83.

Business Insurance. 1985. "Second Opinion Saves NY $2 Million." *Business Insurance* 19(3): 14.

Christofferson, S. M., J. Beeck, N. Baker, S. Hartwell. 1983. *Utilization Review: Past, Present, Future*. Excelsior, MN: InterStudy.

Congressional Budget Office. 1979. *The Effects of PSROs on Health Care Costs: Current Findings and Future Evaluations*. Washington, DC: U.S. Government Printing Office.

Ermann, D. 1988. "Hospital Utilization Review: Past Experience, Future Directions." *Journal of Health Politics, Policy and Law* 13(4): 683–704.

Feldstein, P. J., T. M. Wickizer, and J. R. C. Wheeler. 1988. "Private Cost Containment: The Effects of Utilization Review Programs on Health Care Use and Expenditures." *New England Journal of Medicine* 318: 1310–14.

Graugnard, S. 1987. "Utilization Review System in Preferred Provider Organizations: Performance Versus Promise." *Journal of Ambulatory Care Management* 10(2): 17–24.

Health Care Financing Administration. 1979. *Professional Standards Review Organization, 1978 Program Evaluation*. Washington, DC: Department of Health, Education and Welfare.

——— . 1980. *Professional Standards Review Organization, 1979 Program Evaluation*. Washington, DC: U.S. Department of Health, Education and Welfare.

————. 1991. *Health Care Financing Program Statistics: Medicare and Medicaid Data Book, 1990*. HCFA Pub. No. 03314. Baltimore: HCFA.

Health Insurance Association of America (HIAA). 1990. *Source Book of Health Insurance Data*. Washington, DC: HIAA.

Henderson, M., and S. Wallack. 1987. "Evaluating Case Management for Catastrophic Illness." *Business and Health*, 4(3): 7–11.

Holahan, J., and B. Stuart. 1977. *Controlling Medicaid Utilization Patterns*. Washington, DC: The Urban Institute.

Institute of Medicine. 1989. *Controlling Cost and Changing Patient Care?* edited by B. Gray and M. Field. Washington, DC: National Academy Press.

Kauer, R. 1983. *Evaluating a Corporate Health Care Utilization Review Program: The Case of Deere & Company*. Working Paper #013. Cleveland, OH: Health Systems Management Center, Case Western Reserve University.

Leland, D. A. 1990. "Putting Outpatient Costs on a Low Fat Diet." *Employee Benefits Journal*, (March): 33–35.

Lindsey, P. A. 1989. "Medicaid Utilization Control Programs: Results of a 1987 Study." *Health Care Financing Review* 10(4): 79–92.

Lindsey, P., and J. P. Newhouse. 1990. "The Cost and Value of Second Surgical Opinion Programs: A Critical Review of the Literature." *Journal of Health Politics, Policy and Law* 15(3): 543–70.

McCarthy, E. G., and G. W. Widmer. 1974. "Effects of Screening by Consultants on Recommended Elective Surgical Procedures." *New England Journal of Medicine* 291(25): 1331–35.

National Health Policy Forum. 1986. *The Quality of Health Care: The Peer Review Process and Beyond*. Washington, DC: The George Washington University.

O'Donnell, P. S. 1987. "Managing Health Costs under a Fee-for-Service Plan." *Business and Health* 4(5): 38–40.

Paris, M., E. Salsberg, and L. Berenson. 1979. "An Analysis of Non-Confirmation Rates: Experiences of a Surgical Second Opinion Program." *Journal of the American Medical Association* 242(22): 24–27.

Parks, P. 1983. "Mandatory Second Opinion Programs." *ACS Bulletin* 68(10): 25.

Payne, S. M. C. 1987. "Identifying and Managing Inappropriate Hospital Utilization: A Policy Synthesis." *Health Services Research* 22(5): 709–69.

Poggio, E., H. Goldberg, R. Kronick, R. Schmitz, and R. Van Harrison. 1985. *Second Surgical Opinion Programs: Analysis of Public Policy Options*. National Technical Information Services Contract Report. No. AAI-84-55-VOL-3. Cambridge, MA: Abt Associates.

Restuccia, J. D. 1982. "The Effect of Concurrent Feedback in Reducing Inappropriate Hospital Utilization." *Medical Care* 20.

Ruchlin, H. S., M. Finkel, and E. McCarthy. 1982. "The Efficacy of Second Opinion Consultation Programs: A Cost Benefit Perspective." *Medical Care* 20(1): 3–20.

Rutgow, I. M., and S. Sieverts. 1989. "Surgical Second Opinion Programs." In *Socioeconomics of Surgery*, edited by I. M. Rutgow. St. Louis: C. V. Mosby.

Scheffler, R. M., J. O. Gibbs, and D. Gurnick. 1987. *The Impact of Medicare's Prospective Payment System and Private Sector Initiatives: Blue Cross Experience 1980–1986*. HCFA Grant No. 15-C-98757-50-1. Berkeley, CA: Research Program in Health Economics, University of California.

Shahoda, T. 1984. "Preadmission Review Cuts Hospital Use." *Hospitals* 58(15): 54.

Sloan, F., M. Morrisey, and J. Valvona. 1988. "Effects of the Medicare Prospective Payment System on Hospital Cost Containment: An Early Appraisal." *Milbank Quarterly* 66(2): 191–220.

Sullivan, C. B., and T. Rice. 1991. "Data Watch: The Health Insurance Picture in 1990." *Health Affairs* 10(2): 104–15.

Tyson, T. 1985. "The Evaluation and Monitoring of a Medicaid Second Surgical Opinion Program." *Evaluation and Program Planning* 8(3): 207–15.

Wickizer, T. M. 1990. "The Effects of Utilization Review on Hospital Use and Expenditures: A Review of the Literature and an Update on Recent Findings." *Medical Care Review* 47(3): 327–63.

Wickizer, T. M., J. R. C. Wheeler, and P. J. Feldstein. 1989. "Does Utilization Review Reduce Unnecessary Hospital Care and Contain Costs?" *Medical Care* 27: 632–47.

Wyatt Company. 1991. *The Wyatt Compare™ Database*. Washington, DC: The Wyatt Company.

Zalta, E. 1990. "Managed Care Nemesis." *Business Insurance* 24(8): 43–44.

Zuckerman, S. 1987. "Medical Hospital Spending: Effects of Reimbursement and Utilization Control Policies." *Health Care Financing Review* 9(2): 65–77.

Chapter 7

# Capitation with or without Financial Incentives

Capitated payment, as the name implies, is a fixed "per head" payment to a health care provider for a defined set of benefits over a defined period of time. A provider receives a predetermined amount for each beneficiary prospectively; actual costs of caring for a beneficiary may be more or less than this amount. When actual costs of care are less than the capitated payment, the provider keeps the "profit"; if actual costs are more than the payment, on the other hand, the provider is financially responsible. This payment method in effect merges some of the insurance function with the provider function in that a portion of the financial risk is borne by the provider. The provider may be a health maintenance organization, a preferred provider organization, a hospital, a physicians' group, an individual physician, or another provider. In this chapter we focus primarily on two types of providers: HMOs (which provide the majority of capitated care in the United States) and independent physicians (as a potential model for Medicare).

The incentives for the provision of services that a capitation arrangement presents to an individual physician depend largely on two factors: the nature of the provider and the comprehensiveness of the benefits for which the provider is responsible. Incentives to individual physicians employed by or under contract with HMOs vary according to the specific organizational arrangements. These can be quite different across HMOs and different from the incentives an independent physician might face should he or she accept a capitated payment for an individual patient. For example, an HMO might receive capitation but then pay physicians on a fee-for-service basis. Similarly, plans that require the provider to furnish comprehensive care present different incentives than those requiring only a component of care—such as primary care or care for a specific chronic disease.

Most capitation arrangements are presently accomplished through HMOs, which can be of several forms. The prevailing typology distinguishes four models of HMOs: staff, group, network, and independent practice association. A staff-model HMO delivers care through employed physicians who are under the direct control of the HMO. In a group model, the HMO contracts with one independent group practice to provide services to its enrollees, and in a network model the HMO contracts with two or more independent group practices. In the independent practice association (IPA) model, care is delivered under contract with physicians in independent practice (Hillman 1987).

The growing diversity of HMOs renders this typology inadequate in a number of ways, and alternative approaches to classifying HMOs have been proposed by Welch, Hillman, and Pauly (1990). Although a fully accepted revised typology has yet to emerge, it is generally agreed that at least five dimensions of HMOs can influence their performance and the incentives they present to physicians. These include (1) the method by which physicians are paid for primary care services, (2) whether HMO physicians see HMO patients exclusively or whether they also see patients covered by indemnity insurance, (3) the nature of any financial contract the HMO might have with a "middle tier"—another organization that, in turn, contracts with physicians, (4) the nature of the risk or reward to primary care physicians, and (5) the size and nature of the risk pool used to share the risk or reward. Welch, Hillman, and Pauly's discussion of these dimensions and the incentives they present to physicians is summarized below.

The first dimension, method of payment, typically takes one of three forms in HMOs: salary, fee-for-service, or capitation. Because HMOs often focus cost-containment efforts on gatekeeper physicians (i.e., the physician who determines the level of the care that the patient needs), the financial incentives that each method presents are important. Under both salary and capitation, if physicians provide more services, they simply work harder with no additional income; these methods would thus be expected to exert more control over the volume of services delivered than would fee-for-service. Under capitation arrangements, physicians have an incentive to increase the number of patients under their care, whereas under salary they do not. When the capitation payment covers ancillary services and consultations such that the cost of these services reduces the physician's income, physicians have a strong incentive to control these services; salaried physicians do not.

The extent to which physicians also see patients covered by indemnity insurance is the second dimension that may influence the effectiveness of any financial incentive presented by the HMO. Because a physician may be unwilling to modify his or her practice patterns for a few HMO patients, HMO plans that permit physicians to see non-HMO patients (or that contract with physicians who retain a significant number of such patients) may find their financial incentives less effective than anticipated. The physician who sees other patients simply is not willing to change customary practice for those few patients.

The third factor influencing HMO incentives and performance is whether the HMO contracts with physicians directly or indirectly. Indirect contracting occurs when the HMO contracts with an organization such as a hospital medical staff, a physician group, or an entity formed specifically for payment purposes. This other organization, in turn, contracts with physicians. The HMO may or may not share risk with this middle tier. Because it is the middle tier that contracts with physicians, payment arrangements are not dictated by the HMO (indeed, the HMO may be ignorant of these arrangements). Thus, HMOs that use indirect contracting through a middle tier may have less influence over utilization than do HMOs that contract directly with physicians.

Gatekeeper primary care physicians in HMOs are often encouraged to control utilization and costs through the use of financial rewards or penalties. The use of these rewards and penalties constitutes the fourth variable affecting HMO performance and incentives. Often, a percentage of payment due the physician is withheld during the year and returned only if all or certain costs meet or are below a predetermined target. If actual costs are lower than the target, physicians may be rewarded with a share of the surplus, in addition to the withheld amount. The ways in which HMOs use rewards and penalties will influence their ability to control volume and costs.

Finally, the fifth variable is the number of physicians who are included in the HMO's risk pool. The number of physicians whose practices are considered in deciding whether overall expenditures have met a predetermined target may influence the effectiveness of the rewards and penalties, and thus the overall control of utilization. The smaller the number, the more aware an individual physician will be of the activities of his or her colleagues, and the greater the incentive to modify practice so as to control costs. Larger risk pools, therefore, will generally be less effective in containing service use and costs, when other things are equal, than will smaller pools.

## Capitation in the Medicare Program

The use of capitation as an alternative to fee-for-service payment within the Medicare program became feasible with the passage of the Tax Equity and Fiscal Responsibility Act (TEFRA) of 1982. Regulations for implementing this act were published in 1985, when the program was authorized to enter into risk contracts with HMOs or with so-called competitive medical plans (CMPs), which are private health plans that meet some but not all of the requirements for HMO qualification (PPRC 1988).

The Medicare capitation payment to HMOs and CMPs is based on the estimated costs that Medicare would have incurred had beneficiaries of the plans remained in a fee-for-service system, less a 5 percent savings for the federal government (PPRC 1988). Specifically, an adjusted average per capita cost (AAPCC) is computed for the Medicare enrollee by adjusting the projected per capita fee-for-service expenditures in the HMO's service area for the age, sex, institution, and Medicaid status of the HMO-enrolled population. Additionally, HMOs are required to reduce their Medicare beneficiaries' copayments or increase their benefits if the AAPCC payment exceeds an estimate of the HMO's per capita charges for the remainder of its enrolled population (the adjusted community rate, or ACR, rule). This essentially limits HMO profits from Medicare enrollees to the same level it earns from non-Medicare enrollees (PPRC 1990). These payment rules were intended to distribute the financial benefits of HMO enrollment to the government, the HMO, and the Medicare beneficiary. The government pays 5 percent less than it otherwise would have, the HMO recovers a normal rate of profit, and the beneficiary receives lower copayments, expanded benefits, or both (PPRC 1990).

## Extent of Present Use

Capitation has been used to pay for medical services in the United States since the 1930s, but it was inconsequential as a payment method until its use increased substantially during the 1970s. By 1989, approximately 13 percent of the U.S. population was enrolled in HMOs (PPRC 1990). Thus far, however, capitation has not become a popular option for the Medicare population; currently only about 3 percent of all Medicare beneficiaries are enrolled in HMOs under TEFRA risk-based contracts (PPRC 1990). (The cap on profits might be responsible for this weak supply response.) Further, Medicare HMO enrollment is quite uneven, concentrated in a few large HMOs and in certain geographic areas. One-half of all enrollees are in four HMOs, and 70 percent are located in 14 metropolitan statistical areas (PPRC 1990).

Concerning payment methods, one recent survey showed that 46 percent of all HMOs responding paid primary care physicians by capitation (i.e., a fixed fee per year per patient), 39 percent used fee-for-service, and 15 percent paid salaries (Hillman 1987). The extent to which these payment methods were used varied across model types, however. As would be expected, staff models primarily used salaries (79 percent), whereas only 2 percent of network models used this method. Network-model HMOs responding to the same survey primarily used capitation (76 percent), whereas IPA-model HMOs most often used fee-for-service payment (53 percent).

Capitation payment to physicians is usually restricted to any services provided directly by the primary care physician. However, 40 percent of the HMOs responding to Hillman's survey required primary care physicians to pay for outpatient laboratory tests directly out of their capitation payments or out of a comprehensive fund that included their capitation payment (Hillman 1987). The obligation to pay for ancillary tests out of what might otherwise become their own income reinforces the role of primary care physicians as gatekeepers, or managers of care, within capitated arrangements. Other financial arrangements frequently put the gatekeeper physician at risk for the cost of still other services used by his or her patients. For example, 54 percent of capitated primary care physicians in the HMOs responding to Hillman's survey had a percentage of their capitation withheld in case their use of actuarially budgeted funds for referral to specialists was too high. Some HMOs added further penalties for high referral costs by placing liens on future earnings, decreasing the amount of the capitation payment the following year, or excluding the physician from the program.

Overall, about two-thirds of all HMOs appear to use withholding accounts (Hillman 1987). As would be expected, however, these are most often used when physicians are paid on a capitation or fee-for-service basis, and less often for salaried physicians.

## Rationale for Capitation as a Control on Volume

The conceptual case for capitation as a method of payment that will help to constrain medical utilization and costs is strong. By setting the level of payment per person prospectively, it is true by definition that total expenditures will be affected only by the number of persons at risk, not by variations in the volume and intensity of services provided. The incentives for actual control of costs are robust, because every dollar of cost reduces the provider's net income by a dollar. It is by no means certain that the reduction in volume will come only from low-value services. Capitation could, in principle, reduce the quality of care, the volume of beneficial services, or both. The only unequivocal conclusion is that volume should be lower under capitation arrangements than under fee-for-service payment.

The use of primary care physicians or other professionals as gatekeepers or case managers is an important component of this cost-control strategy, and it may be an important reason for the reduced expenditures in many health maintenance organizations. Cases and services to be managed by the gatekeeper can vary, ranging from primary care only for all patients to all services for all patients (including primary care as well as ancillary services, hospitalizations, and referrals) to selected services for selected patients. In the latter situation, cases can be identified in several ways, such as by diagnosis (i.e., for diseases generally associated with high cost), cost (i.e., case management begins when a threshold of expenditures is exceeded), or procedure (i.e., those that typically result in high cost, such as coronary artery bypass grafting). Although case management systems are often enforced with financial incentives, they might be effective even without incentives because they recommend more efficient practice patterns and recruitment of community resources.

## General Considerations

### Risk spreading and incentives

The incentives produced by capitation depend primarily on the scope of the services to be provided and the nature of the provider. Partial capitation, in which the capitation payment covers something less than comprehensive care (e.g., only primary care), is not likely to be as effective a control on the volume or intensity of all care as is total capitation, because providers would have incentives to substitute noncapitated services for those covered by the annual payment whenever possible (this is discussed in greater detail below). In the case of comprehensive capitation, on the other hand, in which all care must be furnished for the annual fee, providers have much stronger incentives to control overall utilization and costs. Requesting comprehensive capitation from an independent physician (as opposed to an HMO), however, essentially turns the physician into an HMO, a risk that is likely to be too great for an individual physician to assume. Indeed, the extensive administrative infrastructure needed by an HMO to budget properly for services, and the licensure requirements needed to assume insurance risk, suggest that primary care physicians in independent practice are not able to accept such responsibility.

Because capitation puts the provider at financial risk when treatment is provided for severe and expensive illnesses, comprehensive capitation payments to independent physicians, or even to gatekeeper primary care physicians within an HMO who face personal financial penalties for high costs, are particularly problematic. Some of the risk may be averaged over a number of capitated patients, but there remains the possibility of a high-cost patient or group of patients taking up much of the physician's time and reducing his or her real net income. In and of itself, a drastically lower income is simply the mirror image of high exposure to risk. It may become a problem if the doctor responds to higher risk by inappropriately reducing volume. However, because an appropriate volume level is seldom determined, one can only express concern that the financial risk to physicians might become excessive and cause an unacceptably low quality of care to be delivered. Most HMOs (87 percent by Hillman's survey) deal with this problem by protecting the capitated doctor from very high cost caused by outliers. Of course, protecting the doctor financially reduces the incentive to control volume.

The potential remains, under any form of capitation, for a given physician or group of physicians to attract a particularly high-cost group of patients, which can be financially catastrophic for that physician. How serious are the repercussions for doctors (and their patients) who are not engaged in risk pools? Mitchell et al. (1987) aggregated data for Medicare patients by diagnosis and service and found wide variation in the inputs and charges across physicians. It appears that either some physicians treat patients with the same conditions in very different ways, or that average severity varies across physicians in a nonrandom way, with some physicians consistently attracting patients with more serious conditions. These data suggest that substantial heterogeneity is likely to occur across services or patients. However, it can also be argued that, for reasonable values of variance from random factors, physicians who care for the majority of Medicare patients should be able to pool much of the purely random fluctuation over time (Pauly and Langwell 1986). If so, then the finding by Mitchell and colleagues must be the result of a systematic nonrandom distribution of patients by severity across doctors.

Obviously, resolving the question of whether these differences in volume of service among physicians are the result of severity of disease or of patterns of practice is crucial in evaluating the efficiency (and the equity) of capitation. If some doctors treat patients of the same type more intensively than other doctors do, and if this is the variation being measured, then imposing a uniform capitation rate would hurt the former and help the latter. It does not seem inequitable to redistribute real income away from doctors who practice in an especially lavish way, but this would be inappropriate if the doctors who appear to be lavish are actually caring for sicker patients.

Let us suppose, however, that variation in patient severity of illness accounts for the observed differences in volume and intensity. Applying capitation only to new patients would improve equity so long as new patients have or could be made to have a more random distribution of severity of illness. However, if some doctors, nevertheless, consistently attract patients of above or below average severity, then no amount of pooling across doctors could produce an equitable solution, unless severity were built into the capitation payment. With a uniform capitation rate, even grouping a large number of physician recipients would still be expected to yield *net* income differentials within that set, because the doctor who brings costly patients to the pool would surely be less well rewarded, in terms of net income (or income per unit of time worked), than the doctor with low-cost patients. Regulation to prohibit adjustment in net payments would only lead to rejection of the doctor with high-risk patients as a potential pool member.

The only solution to this problem is to develop a way to adjust physician capitation payments for the severity level of the doctor's enrolled population. To ensure access for high-risk patients, such risk-adjusted fees must be developed; there is simply no other way to avoid the disincentive associated with money-losing patients. Raising the capitation rate for all patients will not necessarily solve this problem. Even with very high overall capitation rates, physician income could still be increased further by reducing the number of high-risk patients in the provider panel. Regardless of the capitation level, physicians would be encouraged to search for lower-risk patients, causing serious limitations to access for sicker or higher-risk patients. Alternatively, if certain physicians seem to attract high-risk patients, it might be possible to designate certain physicians to care for those patients under special contractual agreements. This is exactly the same problem Medicare has faced in determining the AAPCC for HMOs, but it is probably a more serious problem at the level of an individual physician.

**Partial physician capitation**

An important alternative strategy could be based on current practice in the Medicare program for end-stage renal disease (ESRD). In this program, the capitation payment for routine services is not intended to cover all of an individual patient's needs comprehensively, only the subset of services related to renal dialysis. Accordingly, nephrologists are capitated only for the routine doctor services associated with dialysis, not for other medical conditions that may arise. In essence, the capitation amount is awarded to a site of care for a specific set of services. Capitation for other types and sites of services, such as home care, rehabilitation centers, and long-term care facilities, could form the basis for determining capitation in the same way.

Implementing partial capitation for care delivered at these sites would be more difficult than in the ESRD program, both for Medicare and for private insurers, because there is no specific condition or service that can be used to identify obviously homogenous groups of patients and because substitution of these services for their alternatives is more likely to occur than it would for ESRD-related services. However, beneficiaries receiving nursing home care might, upon further study, be found to be not much more heterogenous than beneficiaries receiving outpatient dialysis, at least with regard to the need for some subset of services. The common theme among these sites is that the services that patients require are more predictable and routine than all the services a patient might need for any reason.

Suppose for the moment that a physician has been assigned responsibility for caring for a particular set of patients for a specific set of illnesses. (This could in fact be the primary care gatekeeper physician, who manages care for a set of people for the full range of illnesses.) The capitation payment would always cover the range of services the primary care physician provides, but it might or might not include all or part of the cost of other services his or her patients use. It might also involve capitating a specialist for care for a particular chronic condition, as in the ESRD model described above. What are the incentives in this arrangement?

The clearest financial incentive applies to the services that the capitated physician would or could personally provide. If the motivation is to maximize real profit, the physician does that by providing as few services as possible, while still maintaining the size of the patient panel at what is regarded to be an appropriate level. This will probably lead the physician to provide fewer of his or her own services, as well as the other services that are complementary to them, than would be the case under fee-for-service payment, other things being equal. If the gatekeeper must compete with other doctors, including fee-for-service doctors, to retain patients on his or her panel, and if reduced services will cause people to leave the panel, then the difference in service levels between capitation and fee-for-service arrangements will be proportionately less.

What about other medical services that are not complements? In the absence of any risk for the cost of substitute services, the profit-seeking physician under capitation will attempt to substitute capitated services whenever possible. If the services demanded are independent of those the primary care physician typically provides, and if they do not affect the demand by patients to be members of a doctor's panel, the physician will be neutral. He or she will consider only whether the service improves the patient's well-being and will not consider the cost of the service.

Putting the doctor at risk for part of the cost of referred services does encourage consideration of the costs of substitution, but there is no obvious way of guaranteeing that costs to the payer and benefits to patients will be appropriately traded off. For gatekeepers, there will be a greater incentive to increase substitution under capitation than under fee-for-service payment. That incentive can be offset by putting the gatekeeper at risk for some of the cost of substitute services, but then there will be an incentive to provide too little of such services. There is no obvious way to calibrate the incentive to get the volume just right, nor is there any empirical evidence to indicate what the right stimulus is.

With the exception of capitation based on site, partial capitation presents significant administrative difficulties and results in perverse incentives. Given the additional problems of defining what services are at risk and how payments should be divided, partial capitation probably is less attractive to both the private market and to Medicare than is full capitation.

## Other design issues

Another important design consideration is whether, for any given payer and group of enrollees, capitation payment is to be voluntary for patients and doctors, mandatory, or subject to financial incentives. If physician acceptance of capitation is voluntary on a patient-by-patient basis, the issue of self-selection based on expected patient severity is magnified. On the other hand, if capitation is mandatory, the freedom of choice of both patients and physicians is compromised, making the insurance plan less attractive and potentially less competitive (or, in the case of Medicare, less politically acceptable). An intermediate strategy is to offer incentives for accepting capitation as a form of payment, in the same way that Medicare's participating physician program does.

Another possible strategy is simply to make all payment for certain diseases, types of services, or sites of care on a capitation basis, perhaps after a voluntary phase-in period. There are precedents for such a strategy in the public sector. Nephrologists who provide routine physician services to end-stage renal disease patients within the Medicare program were originally paid on a fee-for-service basis, then were permitted the option of capitation for a time, and eventually were all put on capitation. Likewise, Medicaid programs have assigned some beneficiaries to capitated programs. Particularly if mandatory assignment is already imposed, switching physicians to a capitation basis appears to be administratively feasible if it is politically or competitively feasible.

The determination of annual per patient fees is another important issue in capitation in both the private and public sector. The demise of many HMOs during the 1980s was certainly the result, at least in part, of inadequate premiums relative to operating costs. Yet private HMOs must remain competitively priced to attract patients. Similar issues exist within the Medicare program. There the current AAPCC-limited fee for HMO patients is 95 percent of the average cost of patients in fee-for-service plans. But in 1982, 5 percent of patients accounted for 54 percent of Medicare payments, and if a fair percentage of this minority is not treated by the capitated system, then the rates paid to the capitated system are too high (Sisk et al. 1987). In addition, a portion of usual Medicare expenses, such as direct and indirect costs associated with medical education, may not be incurred by the HMO. Increasing capitation levels within the program may thus result in total Medicare expenditures that are higher than before capitation.

## Effectiveness as a Volume Control

### Empirical evidence

Early evaluations of the effectiveness of capitation in containing volume and expenditures suggested that total costs per capita were anywhere from 10 percent to 40 percent lower in capitated plans than in fee-for-service populations (Luft 1980a, 1980b, 1981). These evaluations, however, were complicated by the fact that capitated populations tend to be self-selected and thus potentially healthier than those paying for care on a fee-for-service basis. The RAND Health Insurance Experiment, a randomized, controlled trial of the effect of various insurance plans on the use of services, addressed this self-selection issue (Manning et al. 1984). The results of this study indicated that estimated expenditures for the capitated population were 28 percent lower than for a fee-for-service group that had no cost sharing. The lower cost was caused primarily by fewer admissions and hospital days overall. Because beneficiaries had been randomly assigned to capitated plans, they should not have been significantly healthier (or sicker) than those assigned to fee-for-service plans. Thus, the lower expenditures for the prepaid group would appear to represent true differences in practice patterns between capitated and free fee-for-service plans. The results comparing the HMO with cost-sharing fee-for-service plans in the HIE were mixed, with no overall pattern of significant cost advantage for either method of payment.

In a comprehensive review of the literature on the relationship between payment method and practice, Hornbrook and Berki (1985) report that several studies have demonstrated this lower utilization of hospitals in capitated plans (Luft 1981; Sorenson et al. 1981; Blumberg

1980). They also examined the evidence on costs per service, per contact, and per episode for capitated plans versus fee-for-service plans. They found that costs per patient day and per office visit were not significantly different between the two types of plans, and that little evidence existed of differences in the use of technology. The authors found no studies in which the "typical" bundle of services provided per visit was compared between the two payment methods, and there were no comparisons of episodes of illness either. They did, however, find that members of HMOs do tend to have more ambulatory visits per year. They concluded that substitution of ambulatory care for hospital care is occurring in HMOs, and that it accounts for the overall savings achieved by HMOs. In contrast, analysis of the RAND data casts doubt on the generality of the substitution hypothesis, because lower hospital use was also observed in the cost-sharing fee-for-service plans, but those plans had lower rates of ambulatory care use than did the HMO.

Evaluation of four Medicaid capitation demonstrations showed, during the first year, statistically significant decreases in the use of physician services by adults (either in the percent of beneficiaries with any visits or in the number of visits per user) (Freund et al. 1989). The use of emergency rooms by adults also decreased significantly in all four sites, as did the use of ancillary services in three of four sites. It therefore appeared that capitation did lead to a change in utilization patterns. Because some of the programs based capitated payments on fee-for-service levels from prior years, however, corresponding cost savings were not observed (Freund et al. 1989).

One of the determinants of the effectiveness of capitation is the financial incentive offered to physicians, which is intended to influence their patient care decisions. The experience of the SAFECO Insurance Company's attempt at capitation through an IPA suggests the importance of this financial incentive (Moore, Martin, and Richardson 1983). By using primary care physicians as gatekeepers and putting them at limited financial risk, SAFECO hoped to achieve significant cost savings. In a review of why the program failed in this respect, the most salient fact was thought to be the small financial incentives that were used (i.e., limiting the physician's financial risk to only 10 percent of fees on his or her IPA patients, which typically constituted a small proportion of the physician's practice). The plan removed out-of-pocket cost constraints on enrollees (as most capitated plans do) without imposing significant constraints on physicians (either financial or through utilization review). The gatekeeper function was simply ineffective in controlling costs in that context.

Some have argued that the effectiveness of capitated programs depends more on a group practice effect than on a prepayment effect. Differences between independent practice associations and prepaid group practices in terms of services provided have been indicative of these effects (Scitovsky and McCall 1980; Hornbrook and Berki 1985). The differences may be attributable to the evolution of peer standards within a group and the staffing practices of a group (i.e., a group may not hire additional specialists until the demand is great enough).

Whether capitated plans have been successful in moderating the rate of increase in costs or have simply achieved a one-time savings is also of concern. In 1980, Luft reported his analysis of data from several HMOs and comparison groups over a 25-year period (Luft 1980b). He found that trends in utilization were comparable between the two groups, so that the rate of growth in total costs was only slightly lower for persons in HMOs. An extension of this analysis for the period 1976–1981 confirmed that HMOs cause a one-time reduction in cost but not a moderation of increases in costs over time (Newhouse et al. 1985).

In a more recent review of HMO performance, Luft and Morrison (1991) note that most comparisons of HMOs with fee-for-service plans were performed prior to 1983. Although it is clear, then, that HMOs can achieve lower cost levels than the fee-for-service plans that prevailed in the 1970s and early 1980s, HMO performance vis á vis the more cost-conscious fee-for-service plans presently in existence is not clear.

## Theoretical suggestions about effectiveness as a volume control

If physicians act as patient agents, the financial incentives of capitation will not affect their practice. But capitation may still influence care through its effects on the organization of practice, on professional relationships, and on physician-patient relationships. Reorganization of practice, primarily into multispecialty groups, is often forced by capitation, for example, to take advantage of economies of scale and thus to provide care more efficiently or to share risk across a greater number of physicians. Such organizational effects would likely result in lower overall utilization, even independent of the financial effects.

In a profit-maximizing world, capitation will encourage a physician to attract a large number of patients to his or her panel and then to provide them with the minimal possible level of services. There are likely to be countervailing forces, however, because to attract patients the physician must maintain a level of quality sufficient to maintain his or her reputation and avoid malpractice. To some extent, the level of services provided will depend on the supply of physicians in the local market. If there is an oversupply of physicians relative to the population, and thus competition among physicians for patients, the overall level of services a physician provides will be higher than if there is a shortage of physicians. On the other hand, with a shortage of physicians, underprovision of services would be a real possibility; in this case, quality of care would need to be monitored closely by the payer and patient, or by some other watchdog agency.

Physicians who seek a target income will face slightly different countervailing forces. To attain a given level of income, they will need to attract a certain number of patients to their panels. Assuming that the capitation payment is such that they must see more patients to maintain income, increases in the size of the panels will lead to increases in their work loads. This, in turn, results in less time available for each patient and less leisure time for the doctors themselves. Although there may then be an incentive to decrease the quality of care by spending less time with each patient, quality will also be influenced by the doctors' subjective judgment about their own professional conduct.

The overall effect of capitation on the volume of services in the target-income scenario (as in the profit-maximizing model) will depend somewhat on the relative supply of physicians in the area. If there is an abundance of physicians, the volume of services may actually increase as they attempt to attract patients. On the other hand, if there is a shortage of physicians in the local market (and thus excess demand for their services), there is likely to be an overall decrease in the provision of services. Further, in a situation of excess demand, capitation will likely lead to skimming (i.e., physicians recruiting healthier patients), which compromises access to care for sicker or higher-risk patients. As noted, increasing capitation rates to resolve access problems may actually be counterproductive, because the higher rate means that a target income can be reached by seeing fewer patients, thus aggravating the skimming and access problems.

## Summary and Conclusions

Although analysts have demonstrated that health maintenance organizations are capable of reducing expenditures, principally through a reduction in frequency of hospitalization and length of stay, HMOs have not been shown to moderate the rate of increase of health expenditures over time. The likelihood of capitation having a substantial impact on expenditures will depend in part on the risk arrangement that is implemented, the organization of the capitation programs, and the local supply of and demand for physician services.

The reason that capitation has a constraining effect on volume is not clear. Although some observers believe that physician incentives are important, others have suggested that the group process of physicians working together and the effect of capitation on the organization of practices are the principal influences. It is possible, therefore, that similar changes in practice organization could lead to different practice styles independent of a change in financing mechanisms. Case management may also play a role, though primarily in conjunction with financial controls.

Although capitation has the potential to control volume and expenditures, a number of problems related to capitation make it less attractive than other approaches as a volume control. Empirical evidence suggests that captitation is not associated with moderation in the rates of increase in health care costs, but that it achieves lower costs primarily through a one-time effect. Organizational changes needed to expand capitation significantly beyond the 13 percent of the population currently covered under this payment method may be difficult to realize. Both partial and complete capitation present risk-pooling problems that require case-mix severity adjustments, and the methods needed to perform these adjustments are not well developed. Likewise, either type of capitation requires an equitable determination of capitation fees. Given the current problems with AAPCCs for Medicare HMOs, the failure of so many HMOs during the 1980s, and the significant increases in HMO premiums seen recently, a successful approach to setting appropriate and equitable fees seems unlikely in the near future. Finally, the incentives for underprovision of service presented by capitation raise serious questions about the quality of care under such a system and the need for administratively expensive quality monitoring and control.

# References

Blumberg, M. S. 1980. "Health Status and Health Care Use by Type of Private Health Care Coverage." *Milbank Quarterly* 58: 633.

Freund, D. A., et al. 1989. "Evaluation of the Medicaid Competition Demonstrations." *Health Care Financing Review* 11(2): 81–97.

Hillman, A. 1987. "Financial Incentives for Physicians in HMOs: Is There a Conflict of Interest?" *New England Journal of Medicine* 317: 1743–48.

Hornbrook, M. C., and S. E. Berki. 1985. "Practice Mode and Payment Method Effects on Use, Costs, Quality and Access." *Medical Care* 23: 484–511.

Luft, H. S. 1980a. "HMO Performance: Current Knowledge and Questions for the 1980s. A Research Agenda Considered." *Group Health Journal* 1: 34.

———. 1980b. "Trends in Medical Care Costs. Do HMOs Lower the Rate of Growth?" *Medical Care* 18: 1–16.

———. 1981. *Health Maintenance Organizations: Dimensions of Performance*. New York: John Wiley & Sons.

Luft, H. S., and E. M. Morrison. 1991. "Alternative Delivery Systems." In *Health Services Research: Key to Health Policy*, edited by E. Ginzberg. Cambridge, MA: Harvard University Press.

Manning, W. G., A. Liebowitz, G. A. Goldberg, W. H. Rogers, and J. P. Newhouse. 1984. "A Controlled Trial of the Effect of a Prepaid Group Practice on Use of Services." *New England Journal of Medicine* 310: 1505–10.

Mitchell, J. B., J. Cromwell, K. A. Calore, and W. B. Stason. 1987. "Packaging Physician Services: Alternative Approaches to Medicare Part B Reimbursement." *Inquiry* 24: 324–43.

Moore, S. H., D. P. Martin, and W. C. Richardson. 1983. "Does the Primary Care Gatekeeper Control the Costs of Health Care? Lessons from the SAFECO Experience." *New England Journal of Medicine* 309: 1400–1404.

Newhouse, J. P., W. B. Schwartz, A. P. Williams, and C. Witsberg. 1985. "Are Fee-For-Service Costs Increasing Faster than HMO Costs?" *Medical Care* 23: 960–66.

Pauly, M. V., and K. M. Langwell. 1986. "Physician Payment Reform: Who Shall Be Paid?" *Medical Care Review* 43: 101–32.

Physician Payment Review Commission (PPRC). 1988. *Annual Report to Congress.* Washington, DC: PPRC.

———. 1990. *Annual Report to Congress.* Washington, DC: PPRC.

Scitovsky, A., and N. McCall. 1980. "Use of Hospital Services under Two Prepaid Plans." *Medical Care* 18: 30–43.

Sisk, J. E., P. McMenamin, G. Ruby, and E. W. Smith. 1987. "An Analysis of Methods to Reform Medicare Payment for Physician Services." *Inquiry* 24: 36–47.

Sorenson, A., et al. 1981. "Health Status, Medical Care Utilization and Cost Experience of Prepaid Group Practice and Fee-For-Service Populations." *Group Health Journal* 2: 4.

Welch, W. P., A. L. Hillman, and M. V. Pauly. 1990. "Toward New Typologies for HMOs." *Milbank Quarterly* 68: 221–43.

Chapter **8**

# Expenditure Targets

In the Omnibus Budget Reconciliation Act (OBRA) of 1989, Congress established a mechanism designed to limit growth in Part B expenditures. The mechanism, the Medicare volume performance standard (MVPS), is a type of expenditure target that is designed to work as follows: Each year, after receiving advice from the Secretary of Health and Human Services and the Physician Payment Review Commission, Congress must establish a target rate of Part B expenditure growth. This rate is to include factors such as inflation, newly covered services, increases in the number of beneficiaries, and technological advances. If Part B expenditures exceed this target, then the physician payment conversion factor is to be increased less than would be needed to maintain pace with inflation. If expenditures are less than the target, physicians are to be rewarded with a fee update that is greater than inflation. If Congress does not act on these fee updates with explicit legislation, a default update is triggered. Although the MVPS allows for more congressional leeway than did the originally proposed expenditure targets and includes a floor to the annual fee updates, it is essentially a form of expenditure target. Physicians are enlisted to reduce costs through collective restraint on volume and intensity. Whether volume is in fact restrained or not, total expenditures are controlled. Either volume is limited or the per service price is cut; either way, total expenditure is limited.

Expenditure targets provide a fairly simple approach to cost containment in the health care sector. In the most simplistic form of expenditure targets, the desired level of total expenditures is determined and budgeted prospectively, and spending is simply limited to that amount. What happens if actual charges exceed the target? The difference is recovered either by paying providers only a percentage of their charges per unit or by reducing the overall budget in the next period. Total expenditures are thereby controlled.

In essence, an expenditure target is a predetermined budget for the health services to be provided to a defined population of beneficiaries over a given period—a specification of the total amount that should be spent on health care for that group. Taking into account economy-wide price inflation, the anticipated need for services for the beneficiary population, and the cost and productivity-related characteristics of the technology that will be available for diagnosis and treatment, desired levels of spending can be calculated for upcoming periods (typically one year). By comparing actual total charges at the end of the period to this previously determined target, charges in excess of the desired level can be identified and either not paid or recouped in the next period budget. In their strictest form, expenditure targets cannot fail to control expenditures no matter what the circumstances. Even the modified expenditure targets instituted through OBRA 89 offer Congress control over Part B expenditures that it did not previously enjoy.

Because expenditure targets do not dictate specific practice patterns, they allow greater physician autonomy than some other controls. Compared to utilization management, for example, an expenditure target, because it only needs to affect unit price, leaves the doctor much freer to practice medicine the way he or she regards as best. Compared to the uncertainty about whether other volume-control methods will work at all and which will lead to intrusion into doctor-patient decisions, the certainty and autonomy of expenditure targets should be attractive to both physician and payer.

The use of expenditure growth targets also gives the medical profession a motivating rationale to develop, support, and even implement clear clinical standards and other strategies to achieve lower volumes. Because of the economic consequences of the failure to control volume in an expenditure target system (i.e, lower unit prices for services), physicians would have a strong incentive to monitor practice patterns for appropriateness. Further, the autonomy allowed in such a system would enable physicians to choose the methods by which practice patterns are brought closer to the ideal; these methods could range from informal dissemination of standards in hospital staff meetings to rigorous utilization management.

This emphasis on physician autonomy and the development of clinical standards, along with the guarantee on total spending, was undoubtedly a major factor that influenced the U.S. Congress to include a form of expenditure targets, as opposed to other controls on volume, in the recent Medicare physician payment reforms. Allowing physicians to practice medicine as they see fit, while at the same time controlling the rapidly growing volume of services, is an appealing proposition.

Like all potential controls on the volume of physician services, however, expenditure targets have their drawbacks. Their effects on the appropriateness and actual volume of services is of concern. It is hoped that, faced with a finite budget (as in an expenditure target system), physicians would provide only the most beneficial services, eliminating ones that are only marginally useful or unnecessary. But there is no guarantee that this would happen. Given the uncertainty about the appropriateness of so many medical interventions and the economic incentives individual physicians face in deciding which of several potentially useful services to provide, appropriate as well as inappropriate services may be cut to meet a target. Another possibility is that physicians will be unwilling to care for Medicare beneficiaries if unit prices sink too low, resulting in restricted access to needed services. Finally, because expenditure control is accomplished through adjustment of unit prices, the volume of services can still increase even if total expenditures are constant (although purchasing more services for the same amount of money would not generally be considered a problem). The actual seriousness of these problems would depend on the behavior of physicians in response to price changes, and this behavior is not predictable with any degree of certainty.

Expenditure targets can be designed to cover all services or only specific ones, to allow or prohibit balance billing, and to be mandatory or voluntary for physicians. In this chapter, we focus primarily on a "no balance billing" version that covers all physician services (but not hospital services) for a given population of beneficiaries, in which physician participation would be mandatory. However, because a change in any of these components of an expenditure target would be expected to have significant systemwide effects, each of the other types of expenditure targets is briefly considered as well.

We begin with a brief overview of the use of expenditure targets outside the United States and of their anticipated use in the Medicare program. Next, the three basic elements of an expenditure target mechanism for physician payment—the expenditure projection model, the unit price adjustment formula, and the timing of the price adjustment—are described. After discussing these components of the expenditure target system, we consider the issues that would be raised if balance billing or voluntary participation were allowed. The likely effectiveness, appropriateness, and fairness of expenditure targets as a volume control are then explored, with the three behavioral theories once again used to illustrate the possible effects of expenditure targets on systemwide costs, on physicians, and on the quality of and access to care.

## The Present Use of Expenditure Targets

Although expenditure targets are new to health services in the United States, other countries have had significant experience with them. The Canadian provincial health plans use prospective budgets, with five of the ten provinces recouping excess spending through unit price reductions in either the current or the next year (Lomas et al. 1989). German sickness funds are also budgeted prospectively, with per unit prices determined retrospectively to account for volume in the current year (Kirkman-Liff 1990).

In their 1990 review of the Canadian system, Lomas et al. noted that assessment of the impact of the expenditure targets is premature, because only Quebec and Manitoba had had targets in place for more than three years. Available data for years subsequent to the initiation of the volume controls are consistent with an impact of utilization controls, at least in the short run, but the data are not conclusive. In Germany, the use of expenditure targets appears to have been successful in moderating physician costs. From 1970 to 1978 (prior to the implementation of expenditure targets), physician costs per sickness-fund member increased an average of 11.2 percent annually. Between 1978 and 1987, however, these costs increased only 4.5 percent per year (Kirkman-Liff 1990).

Expenditure targets were implemented for the first time in the United States in 1991, as mandated by OBRA to accompany the Medicare fee schedule. As noted above, each year Congress must set an annual standard for the rate of growth in spending on physician services within the Medicare program (Part B). Comparison of actual growth to this standard, along with other factors, determines the annual update in the resource-based relative value scale (RBRVS) conversion factor (PPRC 1990). For the first time, the rate of growth in physician payment is now influenced by the volume of services provided, with "inappropriately" large increases in volume constraining or perhaps eliminating payment updates in the next year. Congress is partially addressing the potential negative effects of expenditure targets (i.e., cuts in appropriate services) by expanding federal support for research on the quality, appropriateness, and effectiveness of health services, although there is no explicit provision for monitoring quality.

The use of expenditure targets within the Medicare program illustrates the benefit of the greater certainty that this approach to volume control provides. In the past, Congress essentially tried to approximate a target rate of growth in Part B spending by successive rounds of fee freezes and thaws. The proximate rationale for volume performance standards was the fear that physicians might respond to selective or across-the-board reimbursement cuts that could follow the implementation of the RBRVS by increasing their volume—the inducement phenomenon that past experience with price controls suggests could happen. The volume performance standards guard against the possibility that this increase would occur and be so large as to violate the standard.

Volume performance standards together with RBRVS provide an explicit budgetary process for determining what level of increase is appropriate and systematically adjusting average unit prices to achieve it. This greater predictability is an advantage to all concerned, including the Health Care Financing Administration, providers, and beneficiaries.

## Elements of the Expenditure Target Scheme

The three essential elements in an expenditure target scheme are (1) an expenditure determination model, which sets the global budget limit, (2) a unit price adjustment formula, which decreases unit prices when total expenditures exceed the target, and (3) a timing choice, which specifies whether unit prices will be adjusted in the current year (through a partial withholding of payments) or in the following year.

### Setting the target: The expenditure determination model

The expenditure determination model identifies the optimal level of expenditure for the population in question and the desired rate of growth in expenditures, taking into account changes in input prices, desired volume of technological change, and demographic or health changes in the population. Determining the optimal level of health spending is ordinarily a policy or political decision, because there is no objective way to determine what expenditures ought to be. In Germany, for example, the target for any one year is based on the previous year's expenditures, increased by the rate of growth in the wage rates received by the members of the sickness fund (Kirkman-Liff 1990). Normally, future expenditure targets would be forecasted or projected, but it is also possible to make after-the-fact adjustments. Such retrospective adjustments would be particularly useful when unanticipated factors influence the legitimate need for health services—epidemics, for example, or the introduction of beneficial new technologies.

To a considerable extent, the problem in determining the target is similar to that in making or rationalizing any budgetary estimate, such as payment levels for diagnosis-related groups or average adjusted per capita costs for reimbursing health maintenance organizations to meet budgetary expectations. The main difference from DRG pricing, in which prices per unit of service are of primary concern, is that technological changes, input price changes, and changes in the characteristics of the population will also affect the intensity of services provided over an episode of care or during the entire year. This is not as different as it seems, however, because one can view a hospital admission that is reimbursed through DRG payment as a composite of services that can vary in intensity. The DRG price is a projection of the volume and intensity of services needed to provide care to a patient with that diagnosis during one hospitalization. In any event, the need to adjust for technology is the same in projecting the expenditure target and in setting the DRG's prospective rate. The main difference from the AAPCC is that there is no average Medicare benchmark. Here again, the population demographic adjustments are similar.

Some difficult decisions would need to be made to arrive at a tolerable formula. In effect, the formula should incorporate all things that are regarded as "legitimate" reasons for an increase in expenditures on physician services, and should quantify the appropriate amount for the increase. Demographic variables—total number of eligibles, age, gender, marital status—seem like obviously legitimate candidates, and their potential impact on volume could easily be determined from statistical analysis of claims data. The impact of varying illness levels could be quantified in much the same way. Adjustment for input price changes could be based on the Medicare economic index of input prices.

### Accounting for technology

Probably the most difficult task in developing a formula for target expenditures will be judging the appropriate change in technology and the impact it should have on total expenditures. Several factors related to technological change complicate the development of an expenditure determination formula. First, if the expenditure target is for physician services, unanticipated technological changes that shift services from the inpatient to the outpatient setting will trigger short-term problems by causing expenditures on physician services to exceed the target while overall costs remain stable. In the longer run, this penalty on outpatient costs may serve to discourage the development of useful but expensive outpatient technologies, or to impede appropriate shifts from the inpatient setting. On the other hand, to the extent that future technology can be foreseen, cost-effective shifts of this sort can be built into the targets (although this process would be complicated by rapidly developed and disseminated technologies).

Second, a mechanism is also needed to deal with the effect of new clinical standards that have an impact on the utilization of services. For example, if authoritative standards were issued that called for yearly mammography for women aged 40 and older, physicians would be faced with a dilemma: Should they provide this standard of care, knowing that they will be penalized financially when their charges exceed the target? Building desirable or prescribed changes into the target would be necessary, whether or not there are changes in the recommended use of the technology (which could result in upward or downward revision of the target) or in the third party payer's coverage of the technology.

Consequently, a third factor related to changes in technology is that new benefits, mandated by Congress in Medicare or offered in private insurance plans, would need to be budgeted—in the sense that a reasoned estimate of their additional cost would need to be added to the expenditure target. Assurances of fairness would be required for physicians to accept such a control.

Probably the most serious technology-related challenge to determination of an expenditure target is the development of a rational or justifiable process for choosing the rate of annual update. This update determines how much of the new technology that has been developed can be made available for an insurer's beneficiaries. For Medicare, this decision is inevitably (if regrettably) a political one—it will depend largely on overall federal budgetary goals, not on the true value or benefit from new technology. Private insurers would have the perhaps even more difficult task of balancing a more rapidly growing premium against an ability to cover a larger share of new technology.

### The population to be covered

Defining an appropriate population for which a target should be determined involves the usual trade-offs between incentives for limiting services, patient selection, and the risk reduction benefits of pooling. That is, pooling that disperses risk also diffuses individual incentives, because no individual doctor or small aggregation of doctors will gain directly from limiting the services provided. Allowing special targets for certain populations, such as HMOs that have already been established, presents issues of preferred patient selection. Defining the population to be covered under each expenditure target is therefore complex.

As with DRGs, it seems reasonable to calculate different projected expenditures for populations in different areas, but the designation of appropriate geographic areas, as in the case of hospital payment, is not straightforward. Various disaggregations are possible, and several principles should be considered in developing these. First, it must be kept in mind that the expenditures are for beneficiaries, not physicians; thus, a population-based approach is needed. Second, the population covered should be large enough to be administratively feasible and to avoid too many small administrative units. Third, the physician population within a target area should be small enough to allow for peer interaction and influence. Fourth, the size of the area should be one that stabilizes year-to-year variations in expenditures, so as to make the targets predictable. Finally, for Medicare, it would be ideal to use current structures such as existing Medicare peer review organizations to administer the target. Although the objective would be to avoid development of new organizations, that might not always be possible and should not be completely ruled out.

Suppose a target was defined for all physician expenditures in a given county. For all but very rural areas, any random or unmeasurable occurrence of illness would be pooled or averaged enough to dampen any impact of random, individually severe (i.e., costly) illnesses. Measurable systematic changes in illness, such as epidemics, could be built into an after-the-fact adjustment in the target, as could any unforecasted demographic changes. Given appropriate data, important changes in the extent of patient "border crossing" could be detected on a sampling basis. There would be no need to record county of residence for all patients. Pooling over an area as large as a county would also be sufficient to prevent any selection of patients expected to have lower or slower growing medical care costs. Getting the target to be fair is not an insurmountable problem.

It would be difficult, however, to offer serious incentives to control volume if all the doctors in a given (large) county are paid the same amount. The strongest incentives for volume control will work in smaller populations, because the number of doctors may be sufficiently low to offer incentives for, or permit easier coordination of, attempts to limit volume. The cost of better incentives, however, is that the group of doctors would be vulnerable to volume effects of random serious illnesses, and might also be motivated to accept or reject patients for treatment based on the impact they are expected to have on volume. If the geographic areas are defined narrowly, there may also be a greater possibility that one doctor would have patients operating under more than one expenditure target (if his or her "market area" overlaps two different target areas), and that would be confusing. Finally, the administrative difficulties of computing and monitoring many targets would be greater, although a formula approach might ease matters.

On balance, there are considerable risks to making the mandatory geographic areas too small, but avoiding these risks seriously attenuates any incentives. Large areas will make incentives less potent, but areas that are too small will put individual doctors at unfair risk of random serious illness and will increase administrative costs. In the Medicare program, volume performance standards were initially set for the nation's entire Medicare population for both surgical and nonsurgical services; desired rates of growth in spending on most physician services were pooled into these two categories.[1] OBRA 89 also gives the Secretary of Health and Human Services the option to recommend other subnational categories of service for separate volume performance standards; these could be by geographic area, specialty or group of specialties, or type of service (PPRC 1990). As a practical matter, it appears that any feasible populations will be so large that financial incentives to physicians will be eliminated.

One other possibility is a strategy in which targets are defined for an area such as a state or portion of a state, but in which doctors who serve a single population could voluntarily elect to have a separate target defined and monitored for their population (for example, an established HMO). Whether beneficiaries would be allowed to have a say in this matter is an open question, but an equally serious question would be whether preferred risk selection could be controlled. If it could—that is, if the population can be defined so that it is stable and not likely to be selected on the basis of anticipated growth in cost—then such self-designated groups could be permitted. In effect, physicians could volunteer to be subject to incentives to control volume and to receive potentially greater incomes if they succeed in doing so. Note that if populations are defined by the geographic areas in which they live, and targets are defined by a rate of growth from some base level, the HMO problem of preferred risk selection will not arise, unless healthier populations would also be expected to have a lower rate of growth in volume from their lower base.

Private insurers could enact similar expenditure targets for their beneficiary populations, using any of these categorizations to define optimal levels and rates of growth in expenditures. However, using the subnational, even local, populations for expenditure targets fixes the rate of growth on different initial levels of utilization that are difficult to justify. In essence, areas in which volume per beneficiary has been high are allowed to continue to have a higher volume of services even with expenditure targets because they become locked into the high end of interregional variation in volume as a result of the higher baseline.

### *A single target for all services, or separate targets for separate services?*

The other design question is which services should be aggregated. It is possible, although administratively complex, to set different targets for different services and to measure the achievement of such targets separately. (Such an aggregation would be based on type of service, not self-designated physician specialty.) As noted above, this approach is being taken in the Medicare program with the distinction between surgical and nonsurgical services. It could be carried even further, however, to the point of categorizing all cardiac surgery or even all coronary bypass grafts separately.

A sound rationale exists for such an approach. If targets were set for each service and only some services overshot the target, then it would be sensible to adjust prices only for those excessive services. Doing so would also reduce the "inequitable spillover" problem, in which all physicians are penalized for the overuse of a single service or set of services typically provided by a single specialty. One might target a lower (or even negative) rate of growth in volume for services believed to be provided excessively, and yet permit expansion of volume and expenditure for other services thought to be underused. If the Medicare fee schedule had not already introduced relative values, this would be an indirect way of adjusting relative prices closer to an RBRVS or some other relative price schedule (without actually using such a scale) in that it would *automatically* readjust prices for whatever impacts on volume occur. This method of setting targets would adjust prices not according to their input costs as the Medicare fee schedule does, but rather according to the degree of appropriate use. The benefit of developing specific targets for specific services is that, given the uncertain nature of the volume impacts of RBRVS or any other change in relative prices, such a fail-safe limitation on total expenditure might be useful insurance to respond to sizable changes in utilization of certain services.

On the other hand, there are several drawbacks to such an approach. Some authoritative group would need to choose the correct distribution of services (for example, medical versus surgical treatment of coronary artery disease) so that the levels of the individual targets could be set to achieve the desired distribution. However, current knowledge of the relative efficacy of various services is generally not sufficient to dictate a "correct" distribution. Another drawback to service-specific targets is that, over time, using them would distort prices from the RBRVS and would require some correction in the future. Use of a national target with regional practice cost adjustments rather than separate targets allows the work-based methodology of the RBRVS to establish interservice price differences.

## Adjustments in unit prices

The second component of an expenditure target system is the adjustment to be made when actual costs exceed the target. In such a system, deviations of actual from optimal expenditures would cause offsetting adjustments in unit prices. In the simplest one-for-one adjustment formula, increases in expenditures in excess of the target cause reductions in unit price sufficient to hold total expenditures at the optimal level. It would also be possible to have other strengths of adjustment. For example, one-half or some other fraction of excess expenditures due to volume could be captured through the unit price adjustment. There is also a question of whether the adjustment should be one-sided, reducing price for excess volume only, or two-sided, raising price as well when actual expenditures are lower than the target.

On the one hand, a two-sided adjustment would be more equitable if physicians could maintain an acceptable quality of care while becoming more cost-efficient and saving the system money. On the other hand, a two-sided adjustment might provide a strong incentive for underprovision of services (although this effect would be no greater than what occurs in HMOs using financial incentives for control of services). Which type of adjustment to use depends on the amount of confidence placed in the accuracy and appropriateness of the target, as is discussed below.

### Sharing the cost of overruns

A perfectly fixed expenditure target would imply that physicians would share dollar-for-dollar in the cost of overruns (excess volume) and underruns (lower-than-expected volume). Unit prices would fall in overruns but increase in underruns. But things could be made more flexible. Because there may be some uncertainty about whether additional costs are legitimate or not, one could imagine that the insurer would agree beforehand to accept some fraction of the overrun cost. Or there could be a corridor (a percentage of total costs, a fixed dollar amount, or a maximum amount of price reduction) of full physician responsibility for overruns, followed by partial sharing. The size of this corridor could be based on the degree of predictability thought to be obtainable with the formula used, and the details of such an arrangement could be varied to put more or less of the burden of overruns onto physicians or onto insurers.

It may also be possible to quantify the confidence one has in the expenditure determination for any period. The adjustment for appropriate technology, in particular, may be more or less certain, depending on the nature and number of new technologies available. It would be more appropriate for physicians and insurers to share the cost of overruns in times of uncertainty than if the insurer was absolutely certain about the desired rate of improvement in the technology and the associated cost.

Another question is whether underruns—actual expenditures less than projected—should prompt a "dividend" to physicians in the form of higher unit prices. The underrun question is subtle (though perhaps not especially likely): why might expenditures undershoot the target? If the reason is that sometimes there can be good exogenous reasons for spending to grow less than forecasted, then there is no need to share the value of this deviation with doctors. If, however, such underruns actually represent underservice, one could argue for using such an event as a trigger for paying doctors more, if higher fee levels will stimulate a higher volume of services. There is, as we have already noted, some doubt about whether volume responds to price in a positive way, and there may be even more doubt about whether volume growth induced by price increases will occur when and where the underservice occurs. A sensible strategy might be to make the unit price adjustment symmetrical, but to monitor carefully to diagnose the causes of underruns should any occur.

### Timing the price adjustment

The third element of an expenditure target scheme is the timing of price adjustments for excess expenditures. Two methods are as follows:

1. Withhold a percentage of payments until the end of the time period. If there are excess expenditures, distribute only the amount that keeps the total expenditure within the budgeted total.

2. If the target is not met, readjust payment rates for the next period so that, given projected volume, excess expenditures (or a portion of them) will be considered in the calculations of unit prices for the next period.

The first method is frequently used by HMOs to pay primary care gatekeeper physicians, but it has not been used for a total physician budget. It approximates the scheme used by sickness funds in West Germany. The second method has not been used in the United States, but it has been built into Medicare volume performance standards.

These two methods have different implications for physician behavior. Under the withholding strategy, the distribution of the reduction is based on a doctor's past volume, which cannot be changed. Under the other strategy, however, recovering the overrun will alter the price the doctor faces in the next period, allowing the doctor opportunity to adjust volume to the new price. Thus, the price in the next period will necessarily be lower if there is an overrun in the previous period.

Suppose, for example, that doctors expect a 10 percent overrun in period 1 and no overrun in period 2. Suppose also that the nominal price (NP) is to be the same in both periods. Then the expected price that an individual doctor will face under the withholding strategy will be a $0.9 \times NP$ in period 1 and $1.0 \times NP$ in period 2. In contrast, under the "next period" strategy the individual doctor would imagine the net price to be 1.0 in period 1, but he or she would also expect the price for additional volume to be 0.9 in the next period. That is, if every other doctor provided the forecasted volume in the next period and he or she contemplated providing one more unit, the marginal revenue from that unit would be 0.9. Thus, to the extent that volume responds to marginal price (a topic discussed below), the two schemes could have quite different effects on volume in any time period.

### Copayment considerations

Under the withholding method of setting expenditure targets, there would be some ambiguity in determining the copayment for beneficiaries because the final price is not known until total volume is measured. One approach to resolving this dilemma would be to base the copayment on what the unit price would be if volume targets were met, because consumers can hardly be expected to forecast physician volume and adjust their demand accordingly. Using the "next period" strategy, an overrun in one period would lead to lower copayments the next period, which would tend to stimulate demand rather than discourage volume. In this sense, as usual, demand-side incentives and supply-side incentives move in opposite directions. If these lower copayments were felt to be a serious enough problem, it would be possible to base the next period's copayments on what unit prices would have been had there been no adjustment for previous-period overruns.

## Other Design Options: Balance Billing and Voluntary Participation

### Balance billing

In the Medicare program, the use of volume performance standards will combine expenditure targets and balance billing. The structure of the program as planned has already been described: An appropriate rate of growth in total Medicare spending must be projected. If there is an overrun, unit prices are cut by reducing or eliminating fee increases in the next time period. For participating physicians, who have agreed to base their fees on the reimbursement rate (and for nonparticipating physicians whose fees are higher than 115 percent of the Medicare fee, as discussed below), this translates into lower prices for beneficiaries, and lower copayments. Physicians may also agree to accept assignment on a patient-by-patient basis; if assignment is accepted, the (lower) Medicare unit payment is to be accepted as payment in full, except for patient coinsurance.

For a physician who does not accept assignment, the lower reimbursement can mean an increase in prices charged to patients. If the physician continues to bill for the same amount, lower reimbursements by Medicare imply an increase in the balance that is billed. However, OBRA 89 mandates a balance-billing limit of 115 percent of the Medicare fee schedule amount to replace the complex MAAC (maximum allowable actual charge) system, and this limit will be in place by 1993 (PPRC 1990). If the patient does choose to patronize a nonparticipating physician, he or she will be responsible only for the coinsurance and any excess or balance up to the 115 percent limit.

What might be the consequences, under an expenditure target system, of these variations in the amounts patients are charged? The lower coinsurance for services provided on assignment or by participating physicians might cause an increase in patient demand for physician services, because they are less expensive. Whether that demand is satisfied will depend on whether doctors are willing to supply larger volumes; that is, it will depend on how they respond to the volume performance standards. Physicians will face a conflict between what patients want and what Medicare's rules indicate. To the extent that Medigap policies cover the coinsurance, this demand effect will be attenuated.

For beneficiaries who use physicians who do not accept assignment and whose fees are higher than the Medicare fee but lower than the 115 percent limit, the implications are quite different. Suppose actual expenditures exceed projected expenditures, so that the level of Medicare reimbursement per unit is cut. The excess amount charged to beneficiaries will then increase. These charges (which would be in excess of a customary, prevailing, and reasonable maximum) usually will not be covered by Medigap and will result in higher out-of-pocket prices for beneficiaries.

Higher prices for the beneficiary, in turn, are likely to reduce the quantity of services demanded. For profit-maximizing physicians, this decrease in demand will translate into actual volume decreases. Thus, permitting balance billing will generally add a *patient* incentive to reduce volume if overruns are accompanied by increased balance billing. For physicians who do not accept assignment, the effect of a revenue limit will be reinforced. This reinforcement will not occur for participating doctors or those who frequently accept assignment.

The incentive effects of balance billing may not be the most important concern when considering this design option. Instead, the fact that the cost of overruns is shifted forward to patients will be regarded by many as the most objectionable feature. To some extent, this design raises the same issues that are raised by balance billing generally. Could the people who are charged extra use doctors who accept assignment, and do they instead decide to use nonparticipating physicians in order to get some benefit for which they are quite willing to pay? (That benefit might be more convenient access, higher amenity, higher technical quality, better rapport, or snob appeal.) Or are the people who are asked to pay more unlucky, helpless, and without other options?

These questions cannot be answered in this specific context, any more than they can be answered in relation to balance billing. It has been argued that there is some merit in permitting people to override an insurer's judgment about how much expenditures can rise, and how much technology can grow, so long as they know what they are doing and have feasible alternatives. This argument obviously did not persuade Congress when it enacted OBRA in 1989, but the final resolution may depend on what actually happens when the limits on balance billing are in place. It is in principle desirable to make it possible, even easy, for people to supplement whatever their insurance plan, be it Medicare or a private plan, has decided to pay. But it is also important to limit the chances of an unlucky or uninformed consumer being gouged. The best strategy here is probably no different from that for balance billing generally. The insurer should make sure that sufficient acceptable alternatives are available to beneficiaries and should provide strong advice about the availability of those alternatives. Some of the worst excesses could probably be forbidden. But especially with expenditure caps, in which mistakes in forecasting are possible, and in which people may have quite different preferences about what rate of growth they will tolerate, it is probably undesirable to prohibit balance billing and the attendant options it offers to beneficiaries.

What *can* be done is to spotlight and isolate the high-priced providers. Physicians not participating or accepting assignment could be subject to a special expenditure target, say, for just their services. Greater effort could also be made to make beneficiaries aware that these doctors have not agreed with the insurer's judgment about the appropriate rate of growth in expenditures, and therefore should be patronized only with full knowledge that they are different.

## Voluntary participation

The other question to be considered in designing expenditure targets is whether revenue limitation, in any degree of stringency, should be compulsory for all doctors who accept patients covered under a given insurance plan—Medicare or any other. If it is compulsory, an unavoidable consequence is that some doctors may cease to take any patients insured by plans whose prices they feel are too low. The alternative would be to allow voluntary participation in an expenditure target scheme. If the incentive can be made two-sided (i.e., both raising and reducing price in relation to volume), the prospect of higher unit prices for lower volumes could even be a positive incentive to accept such a limit. But voluntary schemes will be less effective at volume control. If insurers are serious about volume control, then they will have to impose some kind of universal revenue limits.

## Effectiveness, Appropriateness, and Fairness of Expenditure Targets

### Effectiveness: A theoretical analysis

There seems to be little reason to doubt the effectiveness of expenditure limits or budgeting schemes in controlling expenditures on physician services. They will work. In the strict expenditure target scheme, whatever volume doctors select, the process automatically adjusts payment per unit so that total expenditures reach the target. In the withholding strategy, the only way to frustrate this control would be to increase volume so much that all the funds withheld would be used up before all services were paid. In the "next period" strategy, volume could conceivably be increased in the next period, but then there would be an even greater price reduction in the period following that. A degenerative process in which price goes to zero and volume goes to infinity is theoretically possible but obviously implausible. At some sufficiently low price, willingness to provide high volumes of services must diminish. Of course, with the Medicare volume performance standard version of the expenditure target, the floor on the reduction of fee increases (that is, no reduction in fees) limits this possibility, except that real fees decrease relative to inflation-corrected dollars.

For those who believe that all physician services are now substantially overpriced relative to cost, an expenditure-targeting approach becomes a politically acceptable way to reduce those prices. With a target, it is not the government's actions, but those of physicians themselves, that reduce the prices that physicians receive.

## *Expenditure targets and "beggar my neighbor"*

If the volume needed to meet an expenditure target at some fee-for-service price level is the volume doctors will, in fact, choose to supply, then the target will be met exactly, the system will be in equilibrium, and total expenditures will be at the proper level. But suppose that the volume at the initial price level is expected by most doctors to be greater than the volume consistent with the target. This means that physicians will expect a price reduction and may be motivated to increase their volume to keep income up. Evans et al. (1988) call this an example of a "beggar my neighbor" policy, with each doctor trying to snatch a larger piece of the total expenditure "pie." Physicians would act out of concern that the price decline that would follow, especially if targets are set on a national or large geographical area level, would lead to prices that are not credible. How serious might this motivation be?

First, because the existence of target-income behavior has not been definitively established, the conclusion that the doctor will want to provide more services at a lower unit price, and that he or she will be able to do so, is far from certain. What we can say is that the process cannot spiral down to zero, because supply at a zero price is surely zero (except for some limited charity service), especially if the price is specific to only one or a few insurance plans and doctors have the opportunity to treat other patients. In a world of foresighted physicians, the price (and volume) will immediately collapse to as low a price as is needed to reach the target level of expenditure. Will that price level be (in)credible—that is, will it be very low? The answer really depends on something we do not know: how far price must fall before the target income motivation to generate demand, if it exists, ceases to have enough of an effect to keep expenditures high. Volume can still increase, but as long as it does not increase more rapidly than price falls, expenditures will still fall. In the West German expenditure-targeting system, prices have not collapsed.

More generally, it is likely that after several iterations doctors would learn their lesson—that volume increases are self-defeating. There would probably evolve (as game theory studies of this issue sometimes show) a "learned parallelism" of strategies that would prevent doctors from offering unbelievably high access and quantity to beneficiaries. In short, expenditure controls would be virtually guaranteed to be a way of controlling spending on physician services and premiums. This process would introduce an element of certainty into budgeting and beneficiary expectations of future premiums.

If, however, physician services are substitutes or complements for other services (including hospital services), there can still be adverse consequences for total spending. Suppose, for example, that some physician services are complements for other services. More doctor visits may mean more drug prescriptions, more lab tests, or even more episodes of hospitalization. If price adjustments cause an increase in the volume of these other services, total costs could be adversely affected. The critical question, then, is whether the prospect of reimbursement limits would cause physicians, individually or collectively, to change the overall volume of their own and other services.

Let us first consider a case in which doctors make volume decisions individually. How we describe behavior depends, as usual, on the behavioral model we assume would be appropriate. Whatever the motivation, in this instance the physician is assumed to consider the economic consequences of his or her action. What will be relevant for financially motivated decisions about volume is the expected additional revenue from providing another service. The best benchmark case is one in which all doctors expect that there will not be an overrun in the current period. Then the nominal or posted price is the expected additional revenue from any service. If that price is consistent with equality between the desired physician volume and the forecasted physician volume, then the expectations will be realized, and the forecast will be met.

Now consider as an alternative the case in which an overrun is expected. This can happen when the volume doctors expect to produce in the aggregate at the current nominal price is greater than the volume assumed in the forecast. The expected additional revenue is the current nominal price minus the expected reduction in price when the overrun occurs. If physicians and patients would respond to lower prices by further increasing volume, as some analysts suspect, then there is a likelihood of aggregate volume increases, even if expenditures will not increase. Of course, the process is critically dependent on how physicians form expectations. If they envision overruns at the volumes that would accompany the initial (high) nominal price, but then understand that price would be cut, they might go on to forecast an even greater increase in overruns and a further cut in prices after the fact, driving the system to the zero price–infinite volume point described earlier.

How the process will actually work depends on how well doctors can forecast what total volume will be. If they can forecast accurately, the process of adjustment can be shortened. A numerical example will illustrate. Suppose the price for the next period is $100. If, at that price, the actual volume is expected to be equal to the volume consistent with the target expenditure level, then the target will be realized. But suppose that all doctors expect that, at a price of $100, actual volume will exceed target volume by 10 percent. Then the price would fall to $90. What happens next depends on forecasts of volume at a price of $90. If, at that lower price, volume is the same as it would have been under a price of $100, then that volume and a price of $90 will occur. In contrast, if volume will be higher at $90 than at $100, physicians would know that the price of $90 will not represent a price that meets the volume target; the price will have to be lower. Physicians know that the price will eventually have to be the price at which forecasted volume and the volume consistent with the expenditure target are equal. Expected (and realized) actual price will automatically jump to exactly the level needed to reach the expenditure target. A similar story holds for volume decline as a response to a lower price, as long as the price adjustment is symmetrical.

In short, with perfect forecasting any expenditure target automatically becomes a self-fulfilling prophesy. It will not even require a period of ratcheting to the correct equilibrium. It may be reasonable to assume, however, that expectations are set in stages, and that physicians will not look beyond the first stage. The process of price reduction would then be an iterative one.

Financially motivated physician behavior may well not be the whole story, however. Setting an expenditure target makes every physician's income depend on the volume decisions of every other physician. For the group as a whole, volume increases do not lead to increases in revenues. Rather, volume changes only serve to alter the shares of a pie of fixed size. Recognizing the financially damaging effects of a volume increase strategy, physicians could collectively take steps to control volume, or even reduce it if price is increased with underruns.

Physicians could collectively try to control the volume of services. Their actual approach would depend in part on the size of the set of beneficiaries for whom targets are calculated. One possibility, although it would require more professional leadership and collaboration than has been witnessed, would be for all physicians across the country to participate in a collective effort to regulate the volume of services provided nationally. It is as possible for all physicians in a given market to develop mechanisms to monitor and sanction themselves as it is for physicians in a specialty to do so. However, notable examples of this kind of professional restraint at the regional, national, or specialty level are few.

To be sure, if a number of physicians are held to a given target, each physician will reasonably ignore the effect that his or her own volume changes will have on the unit price. But the group of all physicians cannot ignore this effect. The smaller or the more homogeneous the group, the easier it should be to organize collective action to do something about it. However, small groups may not have access to the resources that are available to large groups to help them alter practice patterns. They may need to use moral persuasion to encourage other physicians to be conservative in therapy and to avoid services of low marginal benefit. It is possible that some professional self-regulation of volume could emerge in this setting. It is important to note, however, that antitrust issues are likely to arise with any significant sanctions against outlier physicians. For example, antitrust regulation may be necessary to ensure that physicians do not erect additional barriers to deter new physicians who are seeking to establish practices and share in the targeted expenditures. Resolution of these antitrust issues would therefore be critical to effective self-regulation within the profession.

Under the patient agency model of physician behavior, the direct impact of expenditure targets on volume would be minimal. If physicians as agents already provide what they view as optimal care without regard to their own income, the penalties associated with budget overruns would have little, if any, influence on the care they deliver, unless the effect on patients' out-of-pocket expenditures were such that physicians would alter their practices to protect their patients from incurring medical costs. One way to envision a volume effect under this behavioral model is if "low-utilizer" physicians exert pressure on "high-utilizer" physicians (each believes their style of practice is best). In this case, the extent of the volume reduction would be consistent with the mix of high utilizers and low utilizers in the physician population.

## Appropriateness of volume limitations

It is one thing to say that a device will limit expenditures; it is quite another thing to assert that the services then provided will be the most appropriate ones. The recent substantial increase in Part B spending in Medicare is not known to be driven by increases in inappropriate volume, as discussed in Chapter 2. Thus there is an obvious need for a more direct way of determining and monitoring the appropriateness of services, along with any indirect financial device intended to limit expenditures. Insurers, especially Medicare, need to say what they want to buy before they can conclude that any level of increasing expenditures is inappropriate. The obligation to determine a total budget pushes in this direction, but simply setting expenditures at a level sufficient to buy the desired mix and quantity of services does not in itself ensure that those services will be furnished. Someone needs to be equipped with the power and the information to judge appropriateness. That "someone" could be some type of review organization, or it could be beneficiaries themselves. With authoritative advice on defining appropriate services, beneficiaries may be able to come to a judgment about which providers are behaving inappropriately, and which should experience the direct effect of losing customers to whatever administrative sanctions an insurer may impose.

## Fairness of expenditure targets

The most obvious objection to an expenditure target scheme is precisely that it does hold all physicians responsible for the financial consequences of the volume decisions of any one physician. This means that a physician who is making entirely appropriate choices can be punished, in the form of lower prices and income, for the decisions of other physicians with whom he or she is grouped. Because the volume of any one physician with any one insurer is too small to be a reasonable target for budgeting, this spillover is unavoidable. But it is also the incentive for the collective action that may well be the most helpful (and so far unused) way of controlling expenditures. In one sense, expenditure limitation is like a scheme of global capitation for total payment for physician services, but with the capitated revenues still based on fee-for-service fees. The experience of HMOs that have used such schemes would be relevant here but is not generally known. What is known is that such withhold-and-adjust schemes are technically feasible, at least in small self-selected groups of physicians.

A final question is whether it would be more equitable to have an expenditure limitation scheme implemented on a voluntary basis, with physicians agreeing to accept payment in this form in return for a somewhat higher level of unit price. A related question is whether special physician-patient groups such as HMOs or PPOs should be allowed to have a cap of their own. This might be desirable if these groups have already shown themselves to be efficient providers. It does, however, raise the concern that skimming might lead to inequity among providers.

How much insurers should intervene to set such volume controls in place must also be considered. In the Quebec system, there are elaborate—and constraining—limits on the income of each doctor and on changes in volume. West German sickness funds, in contrast, impose fewer special controls on volume, with the view that getting more services for their members for less money can hardly be a bad thing. (Physicians' associations, which administer physician payments, are beginning to implement some controls.) By analogy with Medicare's prospective payment system, it may be appropriate for insurers to limit themselves to setting the appropriate target and the appropriate unit prices, and then leave it up to providers to decide how to react. Trying to impose a set of devices to help doctors cope can be a well-intentioned but counterproductive effort, which puts undue burdens on physicians. Because the fee level eventually gets reduced enough to induce a volume level that meets the target, perhaps insurers can rely on this marketlike arrangement without extensive interference.

## Summary and Conclusions

Because expenditure targets provide predictability and physician autonomy, they are an attractive way to control the volume of physician services. Expenditure targets for future periods could be derived by determining the appropriate growth in aggregate expenditures for a given geographical region over a given time. Expenditure targets would then be defined based on a population of patients, not a population of physicians. If expenditures were to exceed the target, then various mechanisms could be implemented to change fee levels to correct total expenditures either in the current or in the next period. Geographic regions could be established based on the uniformity of input prices, variation in medical practice, the degree to which the physician community would be able to exert influence, and a number of other characteristics.

All three models of physician behavior would predict that an expenditure target would allow insurers to assure beneficiaries that their premiums and the outlays on behalf of their medical care would increase in a predictable fashion (presuming limits on balance billing). Expenditure growth targets cannot fail to control the growth in expenditures. They would enable the medical profession to take responsibility for the control of volume and services and would forge new professional relationships and possibly new physician organizations. For example, peer interaction and review or case management programs, like those in many prepaid practices, might be instituted.

It would be best if physicians were satisfied with the prices to be paid for medical services before an expenditure target system was implemented, so that they would be willing or even eager to participate in such a system. Although there are, at present, perceptions of inequity in reimbursement to physician specialties, the initiation of the RBRVS within Medicare is likely to stimulate a systemwide revision of fees that may mitigate any resistance on this account. Even if expenditure targets are mandatory, they could include certain elements of voluntarism. Within a mandatory expenditure target system, groups of physicians could elect to opt out and to practice within subsystems of the expenditure target population. For example, HMOs or PPOs that have demonstrated their ability to provide care efficiently might choose to be providers with targets for their present populations in order to free themselves from the potentially higher utilization rates of the general physician and patient populations.

A number of design issues exist with regard to expenditure targets, including the method of projecting expenditures, the method of sharing overrun costs or savings, the timing of adjustments, the size of the geographic area, the degree to which assignment would need to be mandatory, the use of balance billing, and the issue of mandatory versus voluntary participation. A number of concerns also exist, including the perceived fairness for physicians who are held accountable financially for the decisions of their peers, the possibility that individual physicians would not limit their own utilization of services, and the possibility that a spiral of increase in volume and decrease in price would occur.

## Note

1. At present, data do not allow identification of certain services (diagnostic radiographs and laboratory services) provided in hospital outpatient departments; thus, these are not included in the MVPS. Certain other Part B services not commonly furnished by a physician or in a physician's office (such as durable medical equipment, ambulance services, and services provided by ambulatory surgical centers) are not included in the MVPS (PPRC 1990).

## References

Evans, R. G., et al. 1988. "Controlling Health Expenditures—The Canadian Reality." *New England Journal of Medicine* 320: 571–77.

Kirkman-Liff, B. L. 1990. "Physician Payment and Cost-Containment Strategies in West Germany: Suggestions for Medicare Reform." *Journal of Health Politics, Policy and Law* 15: 69–99.

Lomas, J., C. Fooks, T. Rice, and R. J. Labelle. 1989. "Paying Physicians in Canada: Minding Our Ps and Qs." *Health Affairs* 8(1): 80–102.

Physician Payment Review Commission (PPRC). 1990. *Annual Report to Congress.* Washington, DC: PPRC.

# Chapter 9

# Service Bundling

The increased volume and intensity of physician services experienced recently has not been associated with an appreciable increase in the number of contacts or episodes of care, at least not in the Medicare program. Taking office visits, hospital visits, other visits, and consultations together, the number of visits per beneficiary per year increased by only 1.4 percent between 1983 and 1986—a time when expenditures per beneficiary grew almost 17 percent (Mitchell et al. 1989). Instead, the recent growth in the volume and intensity of services appears to be the result of an increase in the number and complexity of services per basic unit of encounter—more lab and diagnostic tests per ambulatory visit, for example, or more sophisticated procedures.

Like the other controls, service bundling is intended to discourage physicians from providing services that are profitable but only marginally useful, thereby controlling aggregate volume and expenditures. In this approach, several specific services typically provided at the same time (or for the same episode of care) are "bundled" together as one reimburseable unit. Thus, the surgeon's follow-up visits would be bundled with the surgical procedure itself and all would be paid for with a single sum, with the surgeon deciding how many follow-up visits were appropriate. Payment can also be bundled around a diagnosis: an episode of pneumonia treated in the outpatient setting might be the unit of payment, such that all the laboratory and radiologic exams, in addition to physicians' visits, would be paid out of a sum intended to cover the entire episode of care. The idea is to encourage physicians to provide appropriate care for a finite payment, setting priorities for services in the process.

Three types of bundling, or packaging, have been proposed. *Office visit packages* would base reimbursement on a per visit basis and would include all associated ancillary services for a single visit. *Ambulatory condition packages* would pay for all aspects of a patient's treatment for a predetermined period of time. A lump sum payment would be made to the physician regardless of the type or quantity of care provided. Covered services would include all visits to the physician, all outpatient diagnostic and therapeutic services, and any consultations with other physicians. *Special procedure packages* would combine all services directly related to a given procedure into a single bill and make a lump sum payment to the physician responsible for the procedure. This type of packaging arrangement could be used for all surgical operations, all invasive diagnostic tests (such as endoscopies and cardiac catheterizations), and complex radiologic procedures. It would be appropriate for all locations—office, hospital, ambulatory surgical center, and so on. Special procedure packages would generally, but not always, bundle together the services of multiple physicians.

Actual use of this approach to controlling volume apparently has been limited to the use of global surgical fees that include payment for the surgery itself as well as pre- and postoperative care provided by the surgeon (see Chapter 11). There is no empirical evidence of the effectiveness of such global fees in controlling volume and expenditures. Conceptual discussions of bundling, however, have been presented by Mitchell et al. (1987), Mitchell (1985), and Jencks and Dobson (1985).

In this chapter, we examine first the rationale for the use of service bundling as a control on volume, comparing it with the two extreme methods of physician payment: the per service payment of the fee-for-service system at one end of the spectrum, and "global bundling" of capitation and expenditure targets at the other. Following this we discuss the design of service bundles, first categorizing physicians and services in a way that facilitates thinking about this task and then proposing a set of principles that might guide these bundling choices. Finally, the likely effectiveness of this strategy in controlling volume is addressed.

# The Rationale for Service Bundling

## Incentive neutrality

A useful benchmark for evaluating various physician payment mechanisms is the degree to which they achieve incentive neutrality, a state in which the doctor is financially indifferent to alternative ways of treating a patient (in the sense that his or her real net income is unaffected by the action chosen). The notion is that the physician will then be most likely to choose the action that provides maximum net benefit to the patient. Although incentive neutrality has considerable appeal (implicit in the discussion of RBRVS), it can still allow the provision of very costly services of marginal but positive benefit to the patient, if no lower-cost substitutes exist. That is, in incentive-neutral situations the doctor will not be motivated to resist providing services that benefit patients modestly but at great cost; that is, he or she will not be induced to limit the potential for a "moral hazard."

Incentive neutrality may not occur, however, if patient demand for a service (at a given user price) is less than the amount doctors want (find profitable) to supply. In a situation of excess supply, Medicare could set a lower price. The rationale for the resource-based relative value scale is to address this problem, but there is some doubt as to whether it will do so.

Capitation systems also do not achieve incentive neutrality, because under full capitation there is an incentive to avoid providing costly services regardless of their benefit. To the extent that avoidance occurs, capitation's appeal is lessened, even though it may be more effective than a neutral system in controlling costs.

Neutrality can be relative (as in an ideal RBRVS, before consideration of a multiplier), such that each physician action yields the same positive profit (but there is more profit from more actions in total). Or it can be absolute, such that *any* action and *no* action leave the decision-making doctor with the same real net income. The ideal payment mechanism is one that gets as close to absolute incentive neutrality as possible. Pursuit of this objective will probably not result in as low a level of expenditure as mechanisms such as global capitation that reduce real physician income when additional services are provided (i.e., have negative net marginal income). Pursuit of the less powerful incentive structure represented by neutrality seems appropriate, however, at least until societal decisions about the desired level of intensity of care are made.

## Cost control and institutional feasibility

In the current fee-for-service system, billing codes identify inputs into the process of caring for a patient, but there is no defined output. At the same time, the number of providers (suppliers of the inputs) and the number or types of services each provides are not limited. As a result, insurers pay for the input services without regard to what health care output is being provided, what services are demanded, or whether or not the mix of services provided achieves the output efficiently. Aggregate costs depend largely on the number of providers involved in the process of care and the types and quantities of input services they provide. At current price levels, physicians probably have a positive incentive to expand volume and intensity beyond the level patients would demand were they given accurate advice.

The most comprehensive ways of reducing the cost associated with the total volume and intensity of services (relative to current fee-for-service) are per person, per time period capitation for care and firmly enforced expenditure targets, both of which, to be maximally effective, should cover inpatient and outpatient services provided by physicians and nonphysicians alike. With either approach, payment is independent of the number of providers involved and the amount of service they supply. But these payment mechanisms are drastically different than the fee-for-service system that prevails in this country today, and major changes would be needed to implement them comprehensively enough to have any real effect on overall costs. The institutional structure needed for full capitation to prevent excessive cost limitation, for example, does not yet exist. On the supply side, a complex set of transactions between suppliers would be needed to divide a capitated payment in an efficient way. On the demand side, beneficiaries and policymakers rightly are concerned about the consequences of the strong financial incentives to contain cost that are embodied in capitation and expenditure targets. It is easy to overshoot and go from reduced provision of unnecessary or marginal services to the restriction of services whose benefits *are* worth their cost. These approaches would therefore require effective quality assurance.

As an intermediate step between full fee-for-service and full capitation or expenditure targets, schemes to bundle services in units less inclusive than full capitation (but more inclusive than fee-for-service, with its thousands of different procedure codes) have been considered. The key to the bundling strategy is to identify a "main" unit that approximates or correlates with an output or intermediate good—either an important procedure or an episode of illness—and bundle payment for that unit with the other services that commonly accompany it. The objective is to make aggregate payment less dependent on the number of providers and the amount of input services they supply.

## Defining the Bundle

The main objective of bundling is to control the type or number of services provided. (In theory, incentives for choosing a lower-cost provider, or lower price, for the same service are also present, but here we assume that control of differences in price across providers is accomplished by other means.) The effectiveness of service bundling in reaching this volume-control objective depends in large part on the design of the bundles themselves—that is, on the physicians and services covered by each bundle.

Effectiveness also depends on how physicians respond to the financial incentives inherent in bundling. For example, do they choose a level of services closer to the ideal when they receive no additional income for those services? Compared to the current setting of excessively high prices paid to providers and excessively low prices facing patients, does a system of zero provider gross income and negative net income happen to land closer to the ideal?

We imagine that any "bundled" physician payment system must define major services that are typically accompanied by other services. These could either be specific procedures, such as a colonoscopy, or the batch of services rendered to treat an episode of illness. A particular physician, called the "principal physician," provides this major service and receives the bundled payment.

**Approximations and incentives**

Three categories of services must be considered in designing a bundling approach. *Principal physician services* are almost always provided in fee-for-service practice by the principal physician, if they are provided at all. Examples include follow-up visits and preprocedure evaluations. *Referred services* are typically provided by a physician or provider other than the principal physician, if they are provided at all. Examples would be anesthesia or anatomic pathology services. *Discretionary services* may or may not be performed, and if they are performed, they can be rendered either by the principal physician or by a referral physician. Examples include lab tests and certain procedures such as sigmoidoscopies.

There is a reason for distinguishing these three categories of services. As far as the principal physician is concerned, referred services are generally incentive neutral under current (fee-for-service) pricing arrangements. That is, he or she neither gains nor loses financially by recommending these services. However, there can be financial incentives if there is fee splitting, if the referral physicians are both members of a multispecialty group practice that divides income, if the physician is a shareholder in a service for which he or she refers patients, if the referral leads to an increase in patient satisfaction that results in the patient returning for further care, or if the referral leads to reciprocal referrals from the other physicians. Otherwise, the physician is subject to incentive-neutral prices for such services whether they are bundled or not. In contrast, including these services in the fixed-price bundle means that there is a new economic disincentive against such services. Leaving such services out of the bundle avoids this disincentive (and the fee splitting inherent in it).

The situation for principal physician services is different than for referred services. If price is high enough to generate positive profits for principal physician services, then there is a positive incentive to the principal physician to supply these services under conventional fee-for-service payment, because he or she receives more gross revenue from doing so. If practice costs are not too great, profit will be increased by providing more services. The bundling alternative should then lead to fewer of such services than in a fee-for-service system, because it substitutes a negative incentive for a positive one.

It is the third category, discretionary services, that is the most problematic in a bundling scheme. If the principal physician receives a bundled payment and then refers to other doctors for some of these services, he or she will necessarily engage in fee splitting. At present, fee splitting is a violation of the law in many states, because decisions on whether and to whom to refer should depend on patient well-being rather than on income to the physician. Even if there were no legal concern, dividing payments in this way would require a new set of business relationships among doctors.

There is a trade-off inherent in bundling. If discretionary services are included in a bundle, the principal physician will have a positive financial incentive to refer to the lowest-cost referral partner, if such services are to be performed at all. Yet there is also a strong incentive to avoid providing such services altogether. On the other hand, if discretionary services are not included in the bundle, the principal physician may have an incentive to refer excessively.

Remaining with conventional fee-for-service payment does not necessarily make matters better, however, because the incentives for discretionary services are not neutral under itemized fee-for-service plans either. Principal physicians who are paid on a fee-for-service basis may choose to perform their own discretionary services, as long as there is a positive net income, rather than refer to a lower-cost and more adept referral partner or avoid the services entirely (Pauly 1979).

Some compromise must be sought. A sensible strategy would be one that divides the referral services into two groups based on evidence of whether they are more frequently performed by the principal physician or by physicians other than the principal one. Payment for the former type of service would be included in the package, and separate billing would not be permitted. The latter services, in contrast, could continue to be billed separately. A somewhat different approach would be one based on the comparative cost of (quality-adjusted) services. When the principal physician's cost for some service is close to that of the referral partner, the service could be included in the package. Calculation of individual physicians' practice costs would be quite difficult, however, making this a less practical approach to the division of these services.

## The Basis of Bundling

Is there any reason to choose one of these approaches to combining services over another? Five principles should govern this decision. First, administrative costs of arranging fee division should be taken into account. Second, services provided by the principal physician definitely should be included in the bundle when they are consistently coupled with one another. Third, the more a service is substitutable between the principal physician and other input suppliers, the more appropriate it may be to include the service in the bundle. Fourth, the less the variation in severity of illness that accompanies the major service, the more appropriate it will be to bundle. And fifth, the more likely the services usually provided in connection with the bundle services are to be of low or negative value, the more useful it will be to bundle.

What about a basis for excluding certain related services from the bundle? Are there services that might not need to be included? If some service (other than the major service) provided by the principal physician strongly complements other referred or recommended services, there is no need to include it in the bundle. Its use will be controlled simply because the (complementary) principal physician service is controlled. For example, suppose a medical diagnostic procedure is usually followed by a number of physician visits. Each additional physician visit leads to more diagnostic tests, consultations, and drug prescriptions. One could bundle all these services together, but that would require that the principal physician divide a large payment, and could subject him or her to a large loss of income in the case of a severely ill patient. In contrast, if just the follow-up visits were bundled with the major procedure, the principal physician would not be at as large a risk and would not need to split fees. And yet, such bundling would be as effective as the more inclusive bundling in influencing the volume of complementary services. Because bundling would act to limit the number of follow-up visits, the tests, prescriptions, and consultations that typically accompany these visits would also be limited.

Suppose a primary service can be accompanied by the following:

1. Follow-up visits of variable number, always provided by the principal physician (principal-provided service)

2. Lab tests provided by the principal physician, fixed in number in relationship to the follow-up visits (strong complements)

3. Other diagnostic services, which accompany the follow-up visits about half the time (weak complements)

4. Consultations that are good substitutes for follow-up visits (discretionary services)

5. Home health visits, which are sometimes ordered by the principal physician but which he or she does not provide and which are not substitutes for his or her own services (referral services)

Which services should be included in a bundle? If incentive neutrality is the objective, the home health visits need not be included in the bundle. Because of strong complementarity, there also is no reason to include the lab tests in this example. In contrast, the follow-up visits provided by the primary physician definitely should be included in the bundle.

As stated earlier, the more difficult cases involve those services that are weak complements or discretionary services. The weak complements could be excluded from the bundle under the rubric of incentive neutrality. If, however, it is felt that the volume of these services is sometimes excessive (e.g., if clinical evidence of benefit is present only one-fourth of the time), then they should be included if either the administrative costs to the physician of doing so are not excessive, or if it is anticipated that putting the doctor at risk for the cost of those services will lead him or her to significantly reduce the extent of ordering. The discretionary services, which could be provided by the principal physician or could be referred out, are obvious candidates for inclusion.

Excluding consultations but including services provided by the principal physician will lead to excessive substitution.[1] At least some of the cost of such substitutable referral services should be included in the bundle. One strategy for doing so that would *not* require principal physicians to pay consultants would be to include the cost of consultant services, and perhaps diagnostic tests, as complete or partial offsets against the fee paid to the principal physician. This avoids the need for the doctor to arrange for explicit fee splitting. The insurer would pay directly for the diagnostic tests and consultations and then charge the principal physician based on the level of expenditures for such services. The configuration of such a penalty can be calibrated to focus on behavior that is likely to be inappropriate. For example, charges could be imposed for consultations in excess of some fixed number, and even increased at an increasing rate for larger deviations.

This approach could be used both with services provided by others and with those provided by the principal physician. Suppose that an insurer typically pays $40 for a follow-up visit, and that on average a procedure is accompanied by two follow-up visits but sometimes needs a third follow-up visit. One could reduce the payment for the procedure by, say, $20 for each follow-up visit in excess of two, or else simply pay only $20 for visits in excess of two. In this arrangement, a disincentive to providing the third service is still present, but it is less strong than if a fixed fee per bundle were paid. This strategy would make more sense for services that are sometimes performed by the principal physician and sometimes by others. Or insurers might pay less than full price for such services when combined with a primary procedure, while paying full price for the same test or consultation visit if given in isolation.

Does such a system of penalty charges have as much theoretical appeal as capitation or expenditure targets? At one level, the answer is no. Because the number of beneficiaries in the next time period can be predicted with a sizable degree of accuracy, it would be easier to predict total expenditures and use capitation or expenditure targets. The major argument for a bundling arrangement is that, compared to these other payment mechanisms, it requires less institutional restructuring. It might also be subject to less danger of preferred risk selection, although this is far from certain.

Although the intent of bundling is to decrease the incentive to provide complementary services of low marginal value, bundling could decrease physician willingness to provide highly beneficial services. Surgeons have often been criticized for not providing good pre- and post-operative care, and internists have been criticized for not counseling patients or performing thorough histories. At least part of their reluctance to provide these services stems from relatively low payments for them. Bundling could lead to an even greater reluctance to provide services that are complements to the principal service, and thus could provoke adverse effects on quality. Although this is a potential hazard of any volume control, the incentive to simply not provide a complementary service, rather than to provide it more judiciously, is somewhat stronger with this control.

## The Likely Effects of Bundling

What do the behavioral models suggest about the effects of a bundling strategy? In such a system, the profit-maximizing physician will seek to minimize his or her costs by providing the fewest services possible. Compared to fee-for-service plans, volume will decrease. Quality might improve where there has been overprovision of unnecessary services, but underprovision of necessary services would be a serious concern. There is no reason to expect the single-minded profit maximizer to stop cutting services when the necessary level is reached. If some of the services in the bundle are for referred services and the principal physician is to split the fee, the profit-maximizing physician may choose not to refer and to pocket the referral fee.

The behavior of target-income physicians under a bundling strategy depends on the specific services included in the bundle. If the bundle does include a service typically provided, physicians will need to choose between their professional valuation of the procedure and the possible loss of income caused by providing it without additional reimbursement. Alternatively, the inclusion of a service in a bundle may represent a kind of standardization of practice, and physicians may thus feel compelled to provide an included service even if they have not done so before. The target-income physician can also be expected to induce demand for services not included in the bundle. Thus, overall effects on volume are indeterminate a priori—the volume of some services will probably increase and the volume of others will decrease. Quality may decline if services included in the bundle are not provided or if demand is induced for unnecessary and inappropriate services.

For the physician-agent, the key issue will be the size of the payment for the bundle. If the payment is set just high enough to cover the cost of those services that are optimal (in the sense of benefits exceeding costs), the perfect agent will do the right thing. Too high a price, however, will lead the agent to provide services of positive but small benefit, whereas too low a price will lead to underprovision.

## Summary and Conclusions

Bundled payments do involve less control over total spending than does full capitation or expenditure targets. Not only that, precisely *because* some services are left out of the bundle, there will be an incentive to substitute those services, when possible, for ones included in the bundle. These theoretical defects may be offset by greater feasibility in institutional structure. If arranging that structure is left to physicians, however, this may not turn out to be true. There are some physicians who would have an easy time of it, such as those already practicing in multispecialty group practices. But most physicians are unlikely to be eager to arrange to share fees with suppliers of other inputs to the bundled treatment.

One possibility is for increased bundling to be left as an alternative payment arrangement that a doctor could elect. In return for a payment less than the current average, a doctor willing to serve as principal physician could receive a bundled payment and be able to gain by choosing a more economical mix. To guard against preferred risk selection, it would probably be necessary to require that this option be selected on a participating basis, rather than a patient-by-patient basis.

Bundling is a less aggressive intervention than complete capitation. How are its savings likely to compare with those under capitation? It is worth noting that capitation as practiced by HMOs appears not to have an appreciable effect on cost per episode of care. Instead, savings arise almost entirely by limiting the number of episodes that involve inpatient hospitalization. The key issue is whether bundling would discourage hospital treatment of those episodes of care that accompany the bundled service. Bundling usually does not envision putting the doctor at risk for the hospital charges per se, so it does not provide powerful incentives directed at the one sort of behavior HMOs are known to affect. Some of the other physician services included in a bundle (for example, referrals to consultants) might themselves be complementary to inpatient care, so there might be some effect. However, the primary advantage of bundling is likely to be greater administrative simplicity rather than major cost reductions.

## Note

1. Exactly how much substitution would result would depend on a comparison of the marginal profit for services provided by the principal physician under the old fee-for-service system with the marginal cost of those services, which is the lost profit under a system that bundles all such services.

## References

Jencks, S. F., and A. Dobson. 1985. "Strategies for Reforming Medicare's Physician Payments: Physician Diagnosis-Related Groups and Other Approaches." *New England Journal of Medicine* 312: 1492–99.

Mitchell, J. B. 1985. "Physician DRGs." *New England Journal of Medicine* 313: 670–75.

Mitchell, J. B., J. Cromwell, K. A. Calore, and W. B. Stason. 1987. "Packaging Physician Services: Alternative Approaches to Medicare Part B Reimbursement. Symposium Report." *Inquiry* 24: 324–43.

Mitchell, J. B., G. Wedig, and J. Cromwell. 1989. "The Medicare Physician Fee Freeze: What Really Happened?" *Health Affairs* 8(1): 21–33.

Pauly, M. V. 1979. "The Ethics and Economics of Kickbacks and Fee Splitting." *Bell Journal of Economics* 10(1): 344–52.

# Chapter 10

# Collapsed Procedure Codes

It has been argued that at least part of the recent increase in spending on Medicare physician services is due to something called procedure inflation, which is the practice of billing the same service under a related but more complex code that will result in a higher reimbursement. A system of numeric codes is used to facilitate physician payment. Physicians submit bills to insurers (either directly or through patients) using standardized codes to communicate which services were rendered to the patient. In an attempt to keep the system accurate, some services have been assigned more than one code, each representing a different level of intensity or complexity. Office visits, for example, can be considered minimal, brief, limited, intermediate, extended, or comprehensive and can be provided either to patients new to the physician (making the visit more complex) or to patients the physician has seen previously. Procedure inflation can occur because the more numerous the codes for a service, the easier it is to subjectively rename the service; a brief visit becomes an intermediate one, for example, or an intermediate visit an extended one. This practice might be fraudulent, but because the codes are not explicitly defined, it might also reflect an honest but inaccurate assignment of a code. Procedure inflation, in this context, refers to alterations of procedure codes without changes in the service actually performed.

*Procedure inflation* should be distinguished from "upcoding," which refers to a shift in the mix of services toward more lucrative codes, without evidence indicating whether or not the content of the services has changed. In a study of the effect of Medicare's fee freeze of 1984–1986 on the volume of and expenditures for physician services, Mitchell et al. (1989) noted a shift in the mix of colonoscopy bills toward procedures involving endoscopy beyond the splenic flexure (as opposed to endoscopy stopping short of that). However, there was no evidence offered that this shift in coding misrepresented what was actually done. That is to say, during the period studied it is plausible that the standard of care had shifted toward use of the more complicated procedure. "Upcoding" may represent either procedure inflation or actual high-cost volume expansion.

This chapter focuses on the problem of procedure inflation. Assuming that procedure inflation exists, one approach to controlling the aggregate cost and volume of physician services would be to collapse all codes for a similar service into one or only a few, in a way that retains fundamental procedural distinctions. Payment would then be the same, regardless of which specific service was actually provided, and there would be no incentive to provide or bill for a slightly more complex service. As in other chapters, our consideration of collapsed codes begins with a review of the present use of this approach to controlling the volume of services. We then discuss the rationale for its use and present an analysis of its likely effectiveness in controlling expenditures and volume.

## The Present Use of Collapsed Codes

There has been only limited use of collapsed procedure codes (CPCs) to control the volume of services or expenditures, and virtually no assessment of the effects of this approach on volume or expenditures has been undertaken. In the survey discussed in Appendix A at the end of the book, Medicare carriers reported only using a fairly simple "downcoding" process to counteract the effects of procedure inflation. One example of downcoding is that when the same physician submits two bills for initial visits on the same patient, some carriers automatically record (or "downcode") one of the visits as a follow-up visit. In the same survey, coding changes were reported to be used by only 12 of 120 private insurance carriers. Analysis of simulations of collapsed coding using Medicare data from South Carolina are reported by Mitchell et al. (1987).

## Using Collapsed Procedure Codes to Control Volume

### What difference do labels make?

The doctor knows with certainty what services he or she provided and has opinions and sometimes evidence on the usefulness of those services in a given situation. The patient observes some (though not necessarily all) of the services and may be able to form an opinion about the types of services actually rendered. The insurer observes a bill that is submitted with no knowledge of what services actually were rendered, what the patient's condition was, or what the outcome was. Regardless of the coding scheme, an insurer's ability to detect manipulation of procedure codes is limited.

An insurer's objective with regard to coding is to pay only for those services rendered and to pay the price already determined to be appropriate for those services. The problem is clear: There is no way for an insurer to actually determine what services were rendered or whether they were appropriate. There is always a possibility of some lack of correspondence between what is billed and what should be paid.

It is possible to monitor coding for accuracy. One strategy is to use a system of spot checks to detect and punish specific cases of incorrect coding. From an insurer's point of view, the deterrent effect of any such enforcement policy will depend on the punishment it can impose. An alternative strategy is to monitor the relative levels and changes in frequency of high-revenue codes, and to impose general penalties for unusual changes without regard to proof of specific error. Both strategies impose administrative expenses, and the latter method can be rendered ineffective by gradual and parallel changes in coding.

The doctor must make two fundamental choices when deciding how to deal with a patient who would be a suitable candidate for any of a set of similar services: the first decision is what actually to do for the patient and the second is which service to bill for. Problems arise both in choosing the procedure and in coding it, because the actions the doctor takes may not obviously and automatically match one of the procedure codes under which he or she must bill. The problems, therefore, are of both *choice* and *labeling*. In terms of aggregate expenditures, these translate into problems of (true) high-cost volume expansion and procedure inflation. The use of CPCs would be appropriate in situations in which a physician must bill for one service from a set of similar services, since altering the set of possible procedure codes might solve one or both of these problems.

## The Likely Effectiveness of Collapsed Codes

### Physician behavior and procedure codes

The possible impact and desirability of CPCs depends in large part on how doctors (or their office staffs) decide on the billing code to be used for a given service. But little is known about this process. We therefore begin by considering this behavioral question in the context of a single physician who has the power to direct how his or her services will be billed.

It is important first to distinguish between technical procedures and visits. It seems reasonable to suppose that the actual performance of a technical procedure could be known to the patient and monitored by an insurer. If a physician bills for a fiberoptic colonoscopy beyond the splenic flexure to remove polyps, he or she either did or did not perform this task. Moreover, if there was a polypectomy, tissue would have been removed and examined, resulting in a corresponding bill for pathology services. In contrast, if the physician bills for an intermediate office visit, there is no corresponding set of specific tasks to be performed; the service is defined primarily by the type of patient seen and the type of problem presented. Although there has been some thought given to redefining visits according to specific sets of procedures, at present it would be difficult to judge whether the service really was provided, beyond noting that a visit has occurred.

How does this difference between technical procedures and visits affect billing behavior? Consider first the office visit case. The physician sees a patient for 30 minutes. He or she has seen this patient before in the distant past for a condition possibly somewhat related to the symptoms the patient now reports. Should the visit be billed as limited or intermediate? There is a great deal of uncertainty about which label is correct. If the physician formerly labeled such visits as limited, and now switches to intermediate, we surely could not call that fraud. Neither external observers nor the physician could resolve the fundamental ambiguity about what the label should be. Instead, the reasonable question to ask is what determines how the physician will label the service. We return to this question below.

In contrast, technical procedures have much less intrinsic ambiguity (though there may still be some). Nevertheless, the doctor may in some circumstances choose to mislabel, either for his or her own benefit or for the patient's benefit. (The procedure inflation that increases the level of Medicare payment may also benefit the patient, because the physician who "upcodes" may be more willing to accept assignment.)

The degree to which procedure inflation actually occurs for an individual physician depends primarily on the degree of negative value he or she attaches to fraudulent billing practices. In much the same way as for demand inducement, the doctor might suffer a subjective moral cost from stretching definitions to bill at a more lucrative level. He or she may be willing to move to an adjacent procedure code for which classification might, in any case, be debatable, but may be much less willing to make a larger movement that could clearly be labeled fraud.

The possibility that procedure inflation would be detected (either by the patient or by an insurer's auditing activities) and that penalties would be imposed would also act as a deterrent. The doctor may intuitively attach a subjective (disutility) cost to procedure inflation, with the size of the cost depending on some notion of the distance between what is reported and what was done.

### How will CPCs affect expenditures?

How would a change in the number of technical procedure categories be expected to affect the extent of procedure inflation? We define "extent" as the difference, measured in dollars, between actual billing and the billing that would have occurred had the services been correctly reported. Mitchell et al. (1987, p. 325) argue that "the more numerous the codes for a service, the easier it is to subjectively rename a brief visit an intermediate one, and an intermediate visit an extended one." This statement is obviously true if the alternative is just one code, because there is then no choice. Moreover, if the number of codes is large, it is easier to subjectively rename a simple procedure as a similar but slightly more complex one. So, the rationale is that reducing the number of codes reduces the opportunity for procedure inflation.

There is more to coding behavior, however, than just the ease of renaming. Except for reducing the number of codes to one, any other reduction in the number of codes will *not* necessarily reduce the extent of procedure inflation. Procedure inflation (measured in dollars) might be reduced if the number of codes were cut, but it might also increase. The ambiguity arises for two reasons. First, we do not know with certainty whether (or how) the willingness of the doctor to bill fraudulently varies with the "space" between codes. Second, even if procedure inflation becomes more difficult when codes are condensed in a budget-neutral fashion, the average dollar value of an upgrade will increase, making procedure inflation even more appealing (or at least less unappealing). If the number of codes is halved, the frequency of procedure inflation might fall by half, but if the dollar value of an upgrade to a different code doubles, the net amount of procedure inflation, measured in dollars of aggregate expenditures, remains exactly the same. Reducing the procedure inflation cost thus requires not only that the frequency of upgrading fall, but also that it fall by enough to offset the increase in the cost to Medicare for those upgrades that do occur.

What determines the frequency of procedure inflation? Larger steps between categories presumably make it more likely that an insurer may notice—and punish—the doctor who upgrades codes when billing. Patients are also more likely to notice and raise concern about being billed inappropriately. Finally, the doctor's subjective cost of modifying codes will increase with the size of the step. But, as noted above, although the subjective cost to the doctor increases, the reward for doing so also increases (if reduced coding is budget neutral). Hence, it does not seem possible even to conclude that there will be less procedure inflation.

The real issue is the rate at which physicians are willing to upgrade codes per dollar of financial reward for doing so. If under multiple codes the extra revenue from procedure inflation is less than the subjective cost of doing so, then reducing the number of codes can actually lead to *more* procedure inflation. That is, reducing the number of codes by half will, on average, double the value of upgrading and may well induce more such behavior. Later in this chapter, we will look at some numerical examples that illustrate this point. It may be that "continuous coding" in some circumstances actually eliminates procedure inflation.

If codes are collapsed so that upcoding will be obvious to everyone and penalties will be easy to impose, then collapsed coding will deter procedure inflation. In a sense, the technology of detection and punishment determines how well collapsed coding will solve the problem of procedure inflation. The solution also depends on the true distribution of procedures. If most procedures are in reality clustered about a medium or average procedure, with relatively few truly complex or very simple procedures, then defining three codes—say, simple, average, and complex—will reduce measured volume and intensity. Conversely, if services are distributed near the two extremes, collapsed coding may lead to higher spending.

Detection of upcoding might be enhanced by encouraging beneficiaries to detect and report procedure inflation. Some private insurers have, in fact, instituted programs in which patients are urged to contact the company about bills for services that differ from those provided, on the premise that such coding leads to higher premiums for the insured person. Such education and encouragement might also help in the Medicare program (though the complex nature of Medicare billing could generate many "false positives" that would be costly to investigate). Stronger incentives to beneficiaries would probably be needed, however, to achieve substantial volume effects. One could imagine a process of offering financial rewards (in the form of reduced cost sharing) for reported overbilling. Many patients will, one suspects, be reluctant to report on their doctor, both because of the doctor-patient relationship and because overbilling will, other things being equal, probably make the doctor willing to supply more of the services he or she does provide and, in the case of Medicare, to accept assignment, which is advantageous to the patient.

As with all of the volume controls discussed here, the effects predicted depend on the behavioral model assumed. As is usually the case, patient agents would not be affected by this particular volume control. Profit-maximizing physicians would find their opportunities for inducement changed under collapsed procedure coding, but it is unclear what the new effect would be. If collapsed coding were to reduce the net income per dollar of service obtainable from some procedure or set of procedures, the supply of that service would be expected to be reduced. However, eliminating procedure codes does not necessarily reduce the price received, and the billed volume under profit maximization may be constrained by demand (rather than supply), so that there is no guarantee of lower expenditures. Target-income physicians who face a lower net price because of collapsed coding would respond in much the same way as they would respond to any lower price. The billed volume could either increase or decrease.

## How will CPCs affect volume?

How would moving to CPCs affect *true* volumes of care? Would reducing the number of codes lead to a reversal of volume expansion? The answer depends on the influence such an action would have on both physician-induced demand and patient demand.

### *CPCs and physician-induced demand*

The effect of CPCs on actual volume depends on whether the doctor has an appreciable ability to create demand. If not, then changing codes would have little effect (unless there is excess demand for some services). But suppose the doctor does have some ability to alter the volume of services provided. Moving to CPCs in a budget-neutral way would reduce payment for the high-priced services and increase payment for the low-cost services. (Moving to CPC simply by eliminating intermediate codes might have no effect on net revenues for procedures.) The incentive to substitute services would make doctors less likely to create demand for the formerly high-priced services (whose prices have decreased). But then they *would* want to create more demand for the formerly low-priced services. So, what will happen will depend on how hard it is to destroy demand and how easy it is to create demand for each type of service—something we know very little about. Because the lower-priced services typically require less patient time, one might predict that demand creation for these services would be easier, so that movement to a CPC system would actually increase aggregate dollar volume. But given the present state of empirical knowledge, little more can be predicted.

In fact, the question of how CPCs will affect volume is analogous to asking the more general question of what happens when one changes the relative values for medical services that are close substitutes for each other (i.e., the impact of the resource-based relative value scale). After all, paying the same price for different services in which different amounts of physician time are used contradicts the policy of basing price on relative physician time input. Such a change has no predictable impact on total billed volume; it is as consistent with an increase in volume as with a decrease (see Chapter 11).

### CPCs and patient demand

The introduction of CPCs would change both copayments and balance-billing amounts, typically in opposite directions. As the payment for a service decreases, so too will the absolute amount of the copayment. One would therefore expect an increase in demand for formerly high-priced services and a decrease in demand for formerly low-priced services, exactly the opposite of the expected incentive effects on doctors. Were it not for the high-cost service that has its reimbursement level cut, there might well be an increase in balance-billing. Any increase in patient demand from relatively lower copayments may thus be offset by the higher balance-billing amount. This might be particularly true in the Medicare program, if the introduction of CPCs causes doctors to be more likely to refuse assignment on high-cost services and to accept assignment on low-cost services.

The effect on patient demand of any change in procedure inflation is less clear. If the net effect of having only a few categories is to reduce procedure inflation, and therefore the prices doctors receive, there will also be an offsetting copayment effect. This offsetting effect, which results in lower prices for patients, will stimulate patient demand and increase patient willingness to accept larger volumes of service.

## Summary and Conclusions

Without empirical evidence of the effect of the number of billing codes on expenditures, there is no reason to expect CPCs to slow volume growth. Reducing the number of codes could increase volume; we simply do not know. More generally, if one could monitor to make sure that what is billed is what was provided, it would seem that more, not less, coding refinement would be appropriate. After all, if two services are different in the sense of having differing costs, ideal pricing would require that they receive different prices. Although the RBRVS does not necessarily move toward ideal pricing, its logic would nevertheless suggest that procedures that have different costs would likewise be treated differently. In the meantime, what is needed is more direct study of the empirical effect of the number of codes on reported volume. The variety of systems used by public and private carriers and the frequency of changes in coding should provide a rich set of natural experiments that would answer empirically the question that is theoretically ambiguous.

An alternative to collapsed procedures codes would be to direct efforts at monitoring the services actually provided under current coding, and punishing severely any fraudulent billing. Where there is honest ambiguity about the definition of services (as in the case of visits), it might be well to recognize that trying to measure the unmeasurable is likely to do more harm than good. Paying doctors for visits on a per minute basis, and then monitoring to make sure that the number and length of visits are not excessive, might be preferable. Here again, theory is inconclusive and evidence will be needed.

It would also be desirable to pay careful attention to the introduction of new procedure codes. Permission for a new code should be based on, among other things, a proven ability to monitor the new code and to prevent procedure inflation. It should also be determined whether the new code represents different levels of resource cost than the current alternatives. If cost is the same, defining a new code only generates more opportunity for confusion. Clinical differences between services will also be important.

Collapsing procedure codes can lead to warped incentives for doctors who are telling the truth, and could have a problematic impact on expenditures for those willing to engage in procedure inflation. Although CPCs would save administrative costs and reduce confusion, doctors' frustrations would increase. On balance, it does not appear that CPCs per se can have a major impact on expenditure growth. In essence, collapsing codes in budget-neutral fashion reduces the incentive for procedure inflation by increasing the difference between codes, but this may be offset by the increased incentive to "jump the gap" because of the higher price differential between two codes.

# Appendix: A Numerical Example of the Relation of the Number of Procedure Codes to Total Cost

We have argued in this chapter that the relation between the number of procedure codes and the dollar value of procedure inflation is ambiguous. Under a reasonable set of assumptions about how doctors decide what procedure code to assign, *increasing* the number of available codes would be just as likely to reduce as to inflate Medicare expenditures. This simple numerical example illustrates the possibility that expenditures can be reduced by more codes.

### Assumptions

How much procedure inflation will occur obviously depends on the distribution of services by true codes (the code that is appropriate for the service actually delivered), the closeness of more lucrative codes for any service, and the willingness of the doctor to write down the more lucrative code rather than the true code. The doctor may be unwilling to write down a more lucrative code either because of the possibility of detection and punishment or because he or she feels guilty about stretching definitions too far. We therefore make the following assumptions for this simple example:

1.  Services rated by true codes are uniformly distributed by complexity "units" over an interval from 10 to 30. That is, there are 20 different true services.

2.  Regardless of the number of codes permitted, the price of a complexity unit is $1.

3.  The doctor is willing to increase the stated complexity of a service (compared to the true value) by 0.5 unit for every $1 in additional revenue.

The last assumption is a simple way of specifying a model of the doctor's willingness to upgrade a code. It says in effect that the doctor requires $2 in revenue to upgrade by one unit, $10 to upgrade by 5 units, and so forth. The reason that the doctor would not upgrade for smaller gain could either be because he or she is ethically unwilling to do so, or because the probability of being detected and punished in some way rises at a rate that makes the risk worth taking only for the stated amount of money. This relationship is specified as linear here; it might more reasonably display an increasing marginal cost of upgrading, a possibility that is discussed below.

## Case A: Two prices

Assume that two codes are defined, one at 15 units and one at 25 units, with prices of $15 and $25. Billing for any service is supposed to be set at the closest available code. For example, services of complexity between 10 and 20 are supposed to be billed at $15, and those between 20 and 30 are supposed to be billed at $25. If all doctors billed all services exactly correctly, average expenditures would be $20.

Now suppose that doctors are willing to inflate procedures. Our third assumption implies that services from 15 to 20 will be upgraded to 20. Upgrading a service from 15 to 20 results in a gain of an additional $10, but it requires moving the code 5 units up from its true value. Because one-fourth of all services fall in the range between 15 and 20, it follows that one-fourth of all services are upgraded. Consequently, the average price paid rises to $22.50.

## Case B: Four prices

Let the number of different acceptable codes be increased to four, set at units of 12.5, 17.5, 22.5, and 27.5. In this case, services with true codes from 10 to 15 are to be billed at $12.50, those from 15 to 20 at $17.50, those from 20 to 25 at $22.50, and those from 25 to 30 at $27.50. If procedure inflation occurs, services from 12.5 to 15 are upgraded to 15, for a gain of $5.00. Likewise, services from 17.5 to 20 are upgraded to 20, and those from 22.5 to 25 are upgraded to 25. So, one-half of the services in three-fourths of the range of services are upgraded; that is, three-eights of the services are upgraded for an average gain of $5.00. Hence, the average payment becomes $21.875.

Comparing Case A and Case B, we see that an increase in the number of codes does indeed lead to more procedure inflation, because upgrading becomes easier. But because the gain from upgrading is less, it can happen (and indeed does happen here) that the amount of procedure inflation measured in dollars is less in the case with more codes than in the case with fewer codes. Aggregate expenditures could be cut by adding more codes.

## Case C: Thirty prices

We now assume that there are 30 different codes, one each for the set of 30 services. Upgrading by one unit will only gain $1, not enough to make upgrading worthwhile. Doing more upgrading will not help, because the marginal gain is always less than the minimum gain required to cover the "cost" to the doctor of upgrading.

In this example we get a striking result: if doctors are willing to engage in procedure inflation, the best way to prevent it is to have as many codes as there are different possible procedures. The more codes, the better.

**Summary**

This simple example shows that more codes do not necessarily increase aggregate expenditures. The result comes from the assumption that the marginal cost of procedure inflation by one unit is less than the marginal benefits. So procedure inflation only occurs when there are large jumps in revenue as a result of upcoding, and the size of such jumps is minimized by having many codes. Of course, if the marginal cost of upgrading starts out low and then increases, this conclusion may not hold. But the general proposition—that the determination of whether or not reducing the number of codes will save money is an empirical question, which cannot be settled by theory and does not have an obvious answer—still does hold.

# References

Mitchell, J. B., J. Cromwell, K. A. Calore, and W. B. Stason. 1987. "Packaging Physician Services: Alternative Approaches to Medicare Part B Reimbursement." *Inquiry* 24: 324–43.
Mitchell, J. B., G. Wedig, and J. Cromwell. 1989. "The Medicare Physician Fee Freeze: What Really Happened?" *Health Affairs* 8(1): 21–33.

Part **III**

# Impact of the Resource-Based Relative Value Scale

# Chapter 11

# Volume Effects of Medicare's Resource-Based Relative Value Scale

## Mark V. Pauly

No one is happy with the current method of determining what Medicare will pay toward the cost of physician services. The current customary, prevailing, and reasonable (CPR) system pays different amounts for the same service to different physicians. More to the point, it does not yield price levels that bring forth a set of services we know to be appropriate at costs we know are minimized. Although there are many who believe that the current system is not right, and although it is easy to criticize it, no one is quite sure what would represent a better alternative. One possibility is to have *relative* payments for different services based largely on the amount of time a procedure typically takes, with some ad hoc adjustments for subjectively evaluated complexity and possibly for training time. This approach is embodied in the resource-based relative value system (RBRVS).[1]

This chapter was written by Mark V. Pauly and originally published as "Fee Schedules and Utilization" in *Regulating Doctors' Fees: Competition, Benefits, and Controls Under Medicare*, ed. H. E. Frech III (Washington, DC: The AEI Press, 1991), 288–305. Reprinted with the permission of The American Enterprise Institute for Public Policy, Washington, DC.

The author is grateful to Ted Frech and John Eisenberg for helpful comments. Background research for this chapter was supported by Health Care Financing Administration grant number 99-C-99169/5-01. All opinions expressed are those of the author.

In this chapter, I wish to explore some of the possible consequences of implementing an RBRVS-based system and alternative systems for setting Medicare payment levels. A special concern is the possible impact of RBRVS, and other systems, on the volume of physicians' services of different types. Perhaps not surprisingly, there will be considerable ambiguity about what those impacts will be, and even more ambiguity about whether any given impact can be judged to be an improvement over the current state of affairs. I therefore also explore a kind of "reverse spin" by asking what assumptions about objectives, physician behavior, and patient behavior *would* lead to the greatest likelihood that RBRVS will improve matters.

Doctors may accept Medicare payments as payment in full for 80 percent of their total charge, or they may choose to bill the patient for more than the 20 percent coinsurance. That is, they may accept assignment or may decline assignment. A complex relationship exists between what Medicare pays, the price the doctor receives, and the price the patient pays out of pocket. In the first part of the chapter, I will consider the case of doctors who accept assignment and who sell to patients who do not pay the copayment out of pocket. The effect of RBRVS and other payment policies for doctors who "balance bill" will be treated later, as will the effect of beneficiary payment of the copayment.

## Objectives for the Physician Payment System

The original design of the Medicare payment system was based on the notion that Medicare should reimburse in a way that would just allow the beneficiary to pay the going price in the market for doctor services. That concept has eroded over time, in part because in many markets Medicare is the 800-pound gorilla, unable (even if it wanted to) to leave the market as it found it. In larger part, the gorilla has become more and more dissatisfied with the amount and type and cost of the bananas it is being supplied and has taken steps to unlink itself from a market it feels is not doing what it wishes.

But what is the objective behind physician payment strategies Medicare has tried to pursue? There has been a vacillation between two concepts of what the objectives of payment ought to be. In some respects, Medicare appears to adopt a government contract perspective, imagining that there is some set of medical services it wants to buy (and distribute to Medicare beneficiaries). It wants to buy the right quantity and quality of those services (where quality includes, among other things, "access"), at the lowest possible price.

The paradigm for accomplishing this task is bidding; in an idealized setting, bidding permits a buyer who does not initially know what the lowest cost for some service is or which sellers can produce at that cost to identify both pieces of information.[2] Although real world bidding arrangements may not be perfect, they may be good enough for government work.

The most serious challenge for implementing bidding-type arrangements for Medicare assignment would be the necessity, finally and at long last, that someone specify exactly what it is that Medicare wants to buy. The Health Care Financing Administration (HCFA) would have to take the responsibility of saying how much care is appropriate, for how many beneficiaries, and with what degree of quality and ease of access. Specifying how much implies, of course, that you also say how much is too much, and why.

Once having specified, say, how many lens replacements for cataracts it wants to buy from how many doctors at what locations, Medicare could simply accept the lowest set of bids consistent with this specification. Or, more realistically, the result could be approximated by gradually reducing the current fee levels until the level of services offered, the level of quality, and the conditions of access meet the specified objectives.

In the past, policy makers have frequently suggested that the volume and intensity of care doctors provide for Medicare patients is inappropriately high. It is relatively easy to blame doctors for providing services that are possibly inappropriate, especially when the standard of appropriateness is flexible. It is a much more daunting task for the HCFA to take the responsibility itself for specifying defensible limitations to the aggregate use and quality of care.

Information on the effectiveness of services, which is currently the subject of a great deal of research, is a necessary but not a sufficient condition for implementing a bidding-type system. In cases where bidding would seem eminently feasible and desirable, as in the case of laboratory tests, Medicare has not yet been able to get a system under way. Nevertheless, a bidding system serves as a benchmark of a system that could bring about whatever level of volume and intensity that Medicare desires, and at minimum cost. I will comment later on the possibilities for approximating a bidding system in practice. For the present, it serves as a standard, both for the HCFA and for providers, to which RBRVS or any other system may be compared.

An alternative concept is that the objective of physician payment should be to achieve *incentive neutrality*. Rather than specify particular volume objectives, the notion here is to establish a payment system that yields a physician the same real net income regardless of what types of services are rendered. "Real net income" incorporates both net money income and the amount of time spent performing the service. The idea, then, is that the physician who cares at all about patients will choose the set of services that make the patient as well off as possible, given the knowledge the physician has and given the patient's expressed desires. Put slightly differently, with no distortive financial incentives, the physician will be presumed to act as the *perfect agent* of the patient with regard to volume and intensity, given the knowledge the doctor has of the patient's preferences. Incentive neutrality is less desirable than an ideal bidding system, but it seems to represent the less comprehensive objective of current physician payment policy.

In this sort of system, if it could be achieved, there might be no need for the HCFA to specify what *its* objectives are, since the system would automatically choose what is best for beneficiaries, as based on doctors' undistorted views. The HCFA could then declare victory in the war on Part B costs and pull out of the battle, since henceforth whatever outcome occurred would, by definition, be the right outcome. The problem is that even the incentive-neutral system is not feasible, as the following analysis demonstrates.

## Relative Prices in a No-Demand-Creation World

Let us begin with a simple model of real-income-maximizing physicians who cannot or will not engage in demand creation. Instead, there is a finite quantity that patients demand of each of $S$ Medicare services. Also for simplicity, assume that demands for the different services are independent. The physician is assumed to maximize a "real income" utility function in money income $Y$ and leisure $L$:

$$U = U(Y, L)$$

The production function is given by $Q = Q_M + Q_N = g(W)$, where $W$ is physician hours worked (equal to 24 − $L$ per day), $Q$ is total quantity, $Q_M$ is Medicare quantity, and $Q_N$ is non-Medicare quantity. Let $P_M$ be the Medicare price, and let $Q_N = Q(P_N)$ be the non-Medicare demand curve as a function of the non-Medicare price. Medigap insurance is assumed to eliminate the effect of copayment. We initially assume that all physicians are participating, so that the price Medicare pays determines the price the physician gets. We also initially assume that Medicare demand for any service, though finite, is larger than the amount doctors will supply. Then equilibrium requires that the following holds for every service $i$:

$$P^i_M = \left(\frac{u_L}{u_Y}\right)\left(\frac{1}{g'_i}\right) = MR^i_N$$

where $MR^i_N$, the marginal non-Medicare revenue from service $i$, equals

$$P^i_N + \left(\frac{\partial P^i_N}{\partial Q^i_N}\right)Q^i_N$$

This expression indicates two alternative measures of cost in equilibrium: the (money) value of the leisure that must be sacrificed to produce one unit of service and the opportunity cost of using that time to produce services for non-Medicare patients. The term $(1/g'_i)$ is the marginal time cost per unit of output that Hsiao and others estimate as part of the RBRVS project.[3]

We also need an equilibrium condition across services. We can assume that the money value of a unit of lost leisure $(u_L/u_Y)$ is the same for all services. For every pair of services $i$ and $j$, we then require that

$$\frac{P^i_M}{P^j_M} = \frac{g'_j}{g'_i} = \frac{MR^i}{MR^j}$$

This can be rewritten as

$$P^i_M g'_i = P^j_M g'_j = MR^i g'_i = MR^j g'_j$$

This equality says that Medicare price received per unit of leisure time sacrificed to produce a service must be equal across services, as must marginal private revenue per unit of time. In other words, work time must yield the same net money return per minute in all uses. This is, it should be noted, an *equilibrium* condition; in the long run it *must* hold, and in the short run the system *must* be moving toward it, if the assumptions made in the model are valid. In this equilibrium, price automatically equals cost for any Medicare service supplied in positive amounts; of course, if price equals cost it is also proportional to cost.

Note, however, that this system is implausibly unforgiving. If Medicare should set the price for some Medicare service slightly below the norm, its supply will completely disappear. If it should set some price a little too high, only that service will be supplied. It seems implausible that any real-world government payment system could be that accurate, and yet we do not see Medicare services disappearing from the market. What part of the model must we modify to add realism?

There are two possibilities. One possibility is to adjust some dimension of quality to bring about equilibrium. When Medicare underpays, the content of the service rendered to beneficiaries is adjusted until cost is made to equal price (rather than the other way around). The other possibility is to assume that Medicare beneficiaries are not willing to demand all the services that doctors are willing to supply at the posted prices. Although there is probably some quality adjustment, I suspect that there is currently an excess supply (insufficient demand) for most Medicare services for most physicians. All that excess supply means here is that, if a Medicare beneficiary sought some additional Medicare service, most doctors would be quite willing to render it at current reimbursement levels. I believe that there is such willingness (indeed, eagerness) to supply in today's market. Conversely, if Medicare prices currently do not all bear the same relationship to time costs (the empirical premise on which the whole RBRVS process is built), there *has* to be excess supply for some services, and possibly for all services. With this modification, the new equilibrium statement is that the equilibrium equality condition must hold only for those services for which there is unsatisfied Medicare demand. For the other services, there is excess willingness to supply, and quantity is constrained by demand. We assume that for every physician, there are at least some such "excess supply" services.

Let $P_M^S$ be the Medicare price of a service in excess supply, and $P_M^E$ be the Medicare price of an "equilibrium" service (taking the same amount of time) for which there is excess demand or for which Medicare demand just equals supply. We now analyze the effects on volume of changing $P_M^S$ and $P_M^E$. Suppose $P_M^{Si}$ is reduced for some service $i$ that is in excess supply. As long as the price is not reduced below $P_M^{Ei}$, the conclusion is simple: There will be absolutely no effect on Medicare volume. The only consequence of a price reduction will be to reduce the income (and profit) of the physician. Whether the service is inexpensive or costly, relative to time, there is *no* volume impact. The reason is that, since the price exceeds the amount needed to bring forth enough supply to meet demand, a drop in price, although it may reduce the quantity physicians want to supply, will not cause volume to fall, since demand rather than supply determines volume.

Things are different for changes in $P_M^{Ej}$, the price of a service $j$ that initially is in equilibrium or in excess demand. If the price for such a service is decreased, the volume of the service will unequivocally be decreased, since a doctor who is maximizing net real income will not supply a unit when the price falls below the marginal cost. Supply is constraining. If the price is increased, volume will increase as physicians move along their supply curves—unless demand becomes constraining. Moreover, if the Medicare price cuts reduce Medicare volume, the price in the private market will also be cut, in order to encourage larger amounts of the now more profitable private business. That is, there will be "negative cost shifting." In this case, there need be no concern that physicians will raise prices to others to make up for lower Medicare prices.

These points can be illustrated diagrammatically. We begin with the conventional model of a physician who provides services to Medicare and non-Medicare patients. In Figure 11.1, the physician is assumed to face private demand curves $D(P_1^N)$ and $D(P_2^N)$ for services 1 and 2, respectively. For simplicity, we assume that each service takes the same amount of doctor time and the same level of practice inputs. The conventional model here is one in which the public demand at the price the government sets is large enough to permit the doctor to sell as much as he or she wants of any service to Medicare beneficiaries.

If there were just one Medicare service with price $P_1^M$, and if "$MC$" represents the marginal cost (including the subjective value of lost leisure), the equilibrium is one in which the marginal revenue for each

**Figure 11.1** Effect of Price Changes on Physician Volume with Unlimited Medicare Demand

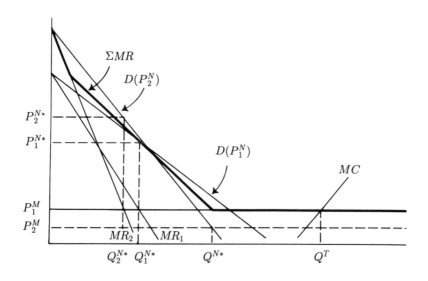

private service $MR_1$ and $MR_2$ is set equal to $P_1^M$. The private prices are those corresponding to those levels of marginal revenue, or $P_1^{N*}$ and $P_2^{N*}$. The total quantity of private services is given by the intersection of a (horizontally) summed private marginal revenue curve (or the heavy line $\Sigma MR$) and $P_1^M$, and the total Medicare quantity is the difference between $Q^{N*}$ and $Q^T$.

Now suppose there is another Medicare service with a lower price (per unit time) of $P_2^M$. The conclusion in the conventional model is straightforward but implausible; the doctor should supply none of this less profitable service to Medicare beneficiaries. He or she should concentrate instead on the more profitable service 1.

To avoid this absurd conclusion, we need to assume that there is a limit to the demand for Medicare services. If the user price is in effect zero, this limit comes from patient unwillingness to accept services that are uncomfortable or time-consuming. Suppose that the limits are $\bar{Q}_1^M$

**Figure 11.2**    Effect of Price Changes on Physician Volume When Medicare Demand Is Limited

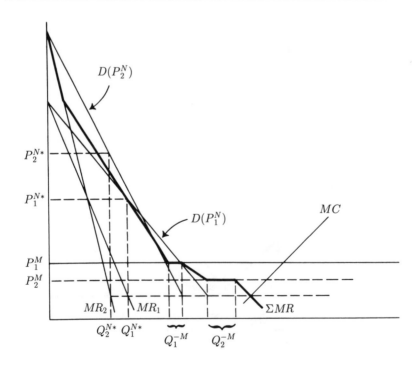

and $\bar{Q}_2^M$ in Figure 11.2. In setting prices and quantities, the doctor moves down the upper segment of $\Sigma MR$ until $MR$ equals $P_1^M$, then produces $\bar{Q}_1^M$ units, resumes movement down the next segment of $\Sigma MR$ until $MR$ falls to $P_2^M$, and then supplies service 2 to Medicare patients. When the Medicare demand constraint on service 2 is binding, the seller moves to the third segment of the $\Sigma MR$ curve and reduces private market price until $MR_1 = MR_2 = MC$.

Now suppose that $P_1^M$ is cut and $P_2^M$ is increased. The overall shape of the $MR$ curve is changed because the segments $\bar{Q}_1^M$ and $\bar{Q}_2^M$ will be moved, but the intersection of $\Sigma MR$ with $MC$ need not be changed. So there need be no change in final private market price or in quantities of Medicare or non-Medicare services. As long as Medicare's prices for both services are sufficiently high, changing those prices has no effect on private prices or on Medicare or non-Medicare quantities; only physician income is affected. The condition needed for this to happen is that no Medicare price falls below equilibrium marginal private revenue.

The message, then, is that if doctors maximize real income and do not create demand, changes in prices serve only to redistribute rents for those services for which $P_M > P_M^E$. They do not affect actual re-source costs, either for physician services or other services that may be complements or substitutes for those services. But for those services for which $P_M \leq P_M^E$, price cuts do reduce volume, and price increases increase volume.

A change in relative prices will have an effect in this model only if it forces price for some service down so low that it falls below the equilibrium price. But the most fundamental point this model makes is a simple one: the main problem with current Medicare prices is not that relative prices are distorted. Rather, it is that virtually all prices are just too high. The simplest strategy is to reduce all prices, regardless of their relationship to cost, and to continue doing so until shortages begin to develop. The least complicated approach would be to begin with current relative prices. Since the quantity Medicare could reasonably desire as appropriate cannot exceed demand, such a strategy moves things in the right direction. Conversely, without getting the overall price level right, there is no obvious particular merit in adjusting relative prices to any specific level.

If beneficiaries do pay coinsurance out of pocket (in contrast with what has been assumed so far), then quantities would rise for services having their prices reduced (for example, surgery) and would drop for the evaluation services having their prices increased. For people who think there should be less surgery, the message from these models will be disappointing: either there will be no change in surgery, or its rate will rise.

## Adding Demand Creation: Justification and Possibilities

It is probably fair to say that the preceding model wholly misses the main rationale behind RBRVS: that is, to offer doctors different incentives in their role as agent/adviser for the patient. And these incentives will matter only if the doctor can and will affect the quantity of services patients receive, that is, if the doctor can and will create demand. In other words, physician incentives will matter only if patient demand does not wholly determine outcomes. The case for RBRVS rests foursquare on the postulate of demand creation. Without demand creation, RBRVS has no economic rationale; its only rationale is a notion of "equity" among doctors. Perhaps more important, its potential effects on volume depend on how changing relative prices will change the amount of demand that doctors are willing and able to create.

The empirical evidence for demand creation is imprecise and contradictory.[4] Demand creation is a flimsy foundation on which to rest a policy of immediate movement to an RBRVS. However "logical" it may seem, the evidence that the doctors will create demand in response to economic incentives has, in my opinion, about a fifty-fifty chance of showing any such effect, much less an effect of practical as well as statistical significance. The foundation of the case for RBRVS rests on a possibly true but unconfirmed hypothesis.

Not only is the empirical evidence weak, but even the theory behind demand effects is ambiguous. The judgments about what volumes of different services *ought* to be provided is, at base, a subjective one. In particular, the judgment that beneficiaries receive too many invasive services and too few evaluation services is still only that, a judgment. But even if one has a view of how one would want volumes to change, there is no theory to tell us unequivocally how to change relative prices to get us from here to there.

What determines whether volume will increase for services for which prices are increased and fall for those for which prices are reduced? The answer, in theory, is ambiguous. The behavioral theory used to understand demand creation is the "sophisticated target-income" theory.[5] This theory imagines that a doctor suffers a subjective utility cost from manipulating information supplied to patients, but is willing to do so, up to a point, for a sufficient financial reward in terms of real net income from selling additional volume. The trade-off between the value of this subjective cost and the value of the financial reward is critical.

The ambiguity in this model comes about primarily because a price change has different theoretical effects on physician incentives to create demand. A budget-neutral cut in price has two conflicting incentives— on the one hand, the physician will want to use fewer of the services that are less profitable than before and more of the more profitable ones. This is a *substitution effect*. That is, as the profit from one service rises relative to another, net money income can be increased by inducing more of the more profitable service and less of the less profitable service. (Note that "more profitable" here is relative to the previous level of profitability; the more profitable service could still be less profitable in absolute terms than the other service.) On the other hand, if Medicare cuts the price on a service that is an important part of the doctor's total business, the price cut will cause income to fall, unless the doctor can increase demand for other services. If income falls, the physician may create demand for the new lower-priced service to get income back closer to the initial (target) level. This is an *income effect*. It is not possible to determine a priori which effect will predominate, and so we cannot determine whether aggregate volume will rise or fall.

Whether a given price change will increase or reduce volume depends on the degree of concentration, in the physician's practice, of the services with increased or reduced prices. The fundamental influence pushing the volume of a service up when its price is cut is an income effect. If avoiding demand inducement is a normal good, there will be less inducement for services of all types if the doctor's total income rises and, conversely, for declines in income.

To take one clear case, if relative prices are changed in such a way that the doctor's income, were he or she to produce the same volume, is unchanged, then we would unequivocally expect the doctor to desire to increase the more profitable services and reduce the less profitable ones. In contrast, if a doctor's practice consists in large part of services with falling prices, the income effect toward more inducement could be strong enough to offset the dampening (substitution) effect of lower profitability. A neurosurgeon, for example, will surely recommend more office visits and other cognitive services for which the relative price rises under the Hsiao versions of RBRVS. But if these services are a small part of the doctor's total income, so that, even after they are expanded, his or her income has still fallen, then the income effect may well cause new demand creation for the invasive (surgical) services.

This is not the end of the story, of course, since consumers may not be willing to accept increases. If fees are raised for office visits, it is not obvious that consumers will be eager to accept doctor advice to make more revisits. And if they do not, then income will fall and it will be less likely that the volume of services for which prices were cut will fall.

Nevertheless, in a budget-neutral world, it remains true that volumes are most likely to move in the expected direction if each doctor's total income does not change much. Rather than redistribute income across specialties, it might be better to make specialty-specific adjustments in relative prices. (This ignores long-run manpower effects.) For instance, a reduction in surgical fees would be accompanied by a larger increase in surgeon office fees than would be true, say, for internist office visits.

But if volumes increase for some services (if in unpredictable ways) in some specialties, will they not fall for others, so at least total Medicare costs will be about the same? Maybe, but maybe not. If the services that have been reduced in price are those that tend to be concentrated in particular specialties, whereas those with increased prices tend to be diffused over all specialties, it is quite possible for aggregate volume to rise. Moreover, total Medicare costs depend not only on what happens to Part B services and expenditures, but also on what happens to complementary Part A services. If invasive procedures are more likely to be associated with inpatient care, and if some such services can rise, there is a real possibility of higher total Medicare costs after a shift to RBRVS in a budget-neutral way.

This is only a possibility, to be sure, and one that I personally would not make my pick if I had to bet on an outcome. But that is precisely the point; given current knowledge and current theory, basing prices on RBRVS is a gamble, with very high stakes.

## Incentive-Neutral Fees

If we cannot tell for sure which direction volumes will follow after a change in relative prices, can we at least describe the set of fee levels we would eventually want to achieve in order to remove incentives for both demand creation and nonprice demand rationing in situations of excess demand? Advocates of RBRVS apparently imagine that getting prices proportional to relative cost is at least arguably a movement in the right direction.[6] Is this necessarily so?

To answer this question, we need to look at what would be a set of incentive-neutral prices. The first point to note is that, for net income to be independent of the volume of any particular services, it is not enough for price to be merely proportional to marginal cost: Price must be equal to marginal cost for each service. Only then will the doctor be virtually indifferent to small changes in volume.

Of course, if prices are equal to marginal cost in this competitive-like equilibrium, they are also proportional to marginal cost. But proportionality alone is not enough. If prices exceed marginal cost in an equiproportional way, that means that the financial incentive to create demand is *uniform* across procedures. But it also means that doctors have a financial incentive to deviate from perfect agency behavior by encouraging more quantity than is in the patient's true best interest.

## Demand Creation: A Best-Case Scenario

There is, in general, no necessary gain from equalizing the incentive to create demand. But is there a special case in which equalizing incentives *does* help?[7]

First, we need to think about the reduction in patients' well-being caused by demand creation and about the physician's perception of that reduction. If the change in relative prices related to RBRVS works as planned, it will even out the incentives for demand creation. More demand, it is anticipated, will be created for evaluation services, and less demand will be created for invasive services. Any demand creation (in the economic sense of demand creation) reduces patient/consumer welfare. The critical normative question, then, is whether the reduction in demand creation for invasive services does enough good to offset the harm caused by more demand creation for evaluation services. Under what circumstances would there be strong reasons to believe that the gains offset the losses?

To answer this question, we obviously have to transform demand creation, in the sense of quantity deviating from the quantity that in truth maximizes the patient's welfare, into a measure of patient welfare. How this transformation occurs depends on how demand creation is limited. Demand creation by doctors can be limited either externally or internally. External limitation has been investigated by Dranove, who imagines that some consumer/patients do detect demand creation and react to it by switching doctors.[8] This behavior in turn limits the amount of profitable demand creation a doctor will undertake.

The alternative model, as noted earlier, is the sophisticated target-income model in which a doctor is assumed to suffer a subjective cost when the "accuracy" of advice deviates from what the doctor regards as the most accurate advice. There are (at least) two interpretations of what generates that disutility. One is that the doctor suffers disutility in proportion to the deviation of actual advice from accurate advice, measured in a technical way.[9] That is, it is the physician's desire to provide technically correct care that imposes the subjective cost. Not doing what he or she was taught is what bothers the doctor. Another interpretation imagines that the physician cares about the level of utility the patient receives.[10] In this case, the doctor must know not only the health consequences of different therapies, but also the determinants of the patient's demand for care, such as income, insurance coverage, and time cost.

Now consider two services that require the same amount of time. Equilibrium in the sophisticated target-income story requires that the ratio of the doctor's marginal profit to marginal disutility of demand creation be equal for the two services. This implies in turn that, if one service has a higher price relative to cost than the other, it will have a higher marginal disutility than the other service.

If only substitution effects matter, and if the marginal disutility to the doctor is simply a transformation of the patient's marginal utility, then there will be a gain to the patient from an RBRVS-based equalization of profit per unit of time. The reason is that a reduction in the price of the high-priced service causes a fall in demand creation, which reduces harm to the patient's utility by a larger amount (at the margin) than the damage caused by the increase in demand creation for the services with increased prices. In short, if the doctor's disutility is the patient's utility, equalizing incentives for demand creation makes sense.

How plausible is this case? I have already suggested that it imposes a substantial information burden on the doctor. If they make decisions only in terms of health effects on patients, then a budget-neutral change in relative prices need not improve patient utility. For instance, doctors may view "hard sell" suggestions for many repeat office visits or benign tests as not harmful to the patient's health. But such services, because of their time cost, may well be of high subjective cost to the patient, higher than the utility cost of invasive services.

Of course, if doctors must guess about nonhealth "costs," but do nevertheless take them into account, this only leads to noise in the prediction about the patient utility consequences of price-induced demand creation. It will still be true that, *on the average*, the marginal effect on patient utility will be greater for services with a high profit.

The approach has a serious implication for procedures rendered to people with Medigap coverage that cannot do harm and that have no time cost. Clinical laboratory tests of specimens already drawn, for example, would fall into this category. Demand for such services will be pushed out as far as is possible. Doctors will, the model predicts, say anything and do anything to get patients to accept such tests. In contrast, the "professional standards" model would not predict that demand would be created to the maximum.

If demand for such "harmless" services is pushed out to the maximum, the implication then is that changing the price doctors receive for those services will, paradoxically, have no effect whatever on their volume, even though there is massive demand creation, as long as demand for those services is independent of the volume of other services.

The most realistic (but most complicated) model would be one that blends these elements. Doctors would take into account the disutility from additional risk to the patient, nonhealth "costs" imposed on the patient, and their discomfort at deviation from what they regard as best practice, and would trade all of this off against the additional net revenue from creating demand. Then the critical factor in determining whether high-priced services that carry high physician disutility from demand creation are also services of high patient disutility is the relative importance of those concerns. The most likely outcome, of course, is that this mixture varies across services. Not all higher-profit services will be doing more marginal damage than all lower-profit services, even though on average marginal damage is positively related to profit.

What is needed is obviously better empirical information on patient utility and the reasons behind doctor motivation for demand creation (which, remember, may not exist at all). We know little about the former and nothing about the latter. In the interim, changing relative prices to equalize profitability has a chance to do some good, and is unlikely to do harm on average. But an empirically based, carefully monitored program that investigates the consequences of a variety of changes in relative prices is much superior to a program that does something for the sake of doing something because there is pressure for "effective" action, regardless of what the effect will actually be.

## Modifications to the Basic Model

The basic model can be modified in two ways: (1) by asking whether a reduction in price can ever cause an increase in volume in a no-demand-creation model with services that mix demand and supply constraints; and (2) by considering the effect of changes in relative prices when some doctors do not accept assignment or do not participate.

Suppose that when the price of a specific service is reduced it drops below the level at which demand can be satisfied. For some doctors, the service is now "unprofitable," given the opportunity cost in terms of lost private-sector revenues or lost leisure. Suppose too that other services that are rendered to patients who seek this service are also demand-constrained. Relative to the preferred service, these services may be too time-consuming, too costly, too uncomfortable, or even too dangerous for patients to accept, but they do carry positive marginal profits (as do all demand-constrained services).

Changing what Medicare pays by cutting price for some specific service may then alter the implicit arrangement between provider and patient as follows. In return for agreeing to accept more of the services that impose too high a time, discomfort, or risk cost, the patient will be provided with the now unprofitable preferred service. In effect, patient and doctor agree to a set of services that extract more revenue and more profit from Medicare.

In reality, the bargaining will obviously not be so overt. Instead, the arrangement will probably become part of the package of services a physician offers to all patients, as his or her preferred style of care. The change can also be seen as a substitution of a higher time cost form of the service. The critical point is that this sort of "demand inducement" is not in any way inconsistent with a neoclassical model of physician supply. No manipulation of information, and no patient ignorance is involved; patients *gain* from this change, in comparison with the only other feasible alternative of no care from this physician. In effect, the provider response to Medicare's reduction in what it pays is to shift cost to the patient, not in the form of higher money cost (since that is ruled out by the assumption that assignment is accepted), but in the form of higher nonmonetary cost.

What will happen in a no-demand-creation model if the doctor does *not* accept assignment and relative Medicare fees are changed? To answer this question fully, one would need a model of the decision to accept assignment and the decision to set the gross price. For a doctor who is already declining assignment but who has the ability to raise his or her gross price, the immediate consequence is obvious: a cut in what Medicare pays will increase the amount the patient is balance-billed (even if the gross price falls a little). Since Medigap does not usually cover all charges in excess of the Medicare reasonable charge, the net effect of an increase in user price is likely to be a decrease in quantity demanded, to accompany this shifting of money cost to the beneficiary. Because the gross price falls, the doctor will also wish to reduce the quantity of services delivered to Medicare patients, since those services will now be less profitable than services rendered to private patients. It is just that the gross price will not fall dollar for dollar in response to a cut in Medicare payments; this is where no assignment differs from the assignment case.

The normative evaluation of this case under the neoclassical no-demand-creation assumption is therefore relatively straightforward. As Medicare pays less for some service, it causes costs to be shifted to the consumers of the service; conversely, increases in payments for other services make consumers of those services better off. A balanced-budget change in relative reimbursements therefore helps some beneficiaries (those who will consume the price-increased services) and hurts others (those who will consume the price-reduced services). Without more information, it is impossible on economic grounds to tell which state is preferable. We can say, however, that there is no particular rationale for the shift to new relative prices, just as there is no rationale against it.

In contrast to the assignment case, the "demand effect" on what patients want is larger, and the supply effect on what doctors want is smaller. In a regime of excess supply, there could be a larger effect on volume for balance-billed services than for services for which assignment is accepted. But, here again, the main conclusion has to be that we do not know enough to make even reasonable guesses.

## Conclusion

There is a good chance that movement to a resource-based system of relative prices will, after a great deal of sound and fury, signify nothing except a redistribution of monopoly rents or quasi rents among doctors. There may eventually be a change in the specialty choices of physicians, but the most likely short-run response, in the models examined in this chapter, is little or no change in aggregate expenditures or in service volumes.

This prediction is surrounded by enormous variance, however. Depending on a host of unknowns (How important is the effect of relative prices on doctor desire and ability to create or destroy demand? How concentrated will relative price changes be across practices? and, What will happen to the nonmonetary price patients pay?), things could change drastically, but in wholly unpredictable ways. There is a possibility that net patient utility will increase, but no guarantee here, either.

It is not clear that there is anything terribly broken about how Medicare sets doctors' payments that we know how to fix by jiggling relative prices. The de facto payment limitation in the current arrangement which RBRVS will replace (as most physicians are bound by the prevailing charge limit) means that the charge that this older system is inflationary is no longer true. The current system is, for the great majority of doctors, a fee schedule. It does have the virtue of familiarity, but the defect of complexity. Just as "an old tax is a good tax," so an old level of relative payments, because providers have adjusted to it, may well beat the consternation that radical change will cause; on the other hand, an old tax or an old payment method that no one understands may not be so desirable after all.

The current pattern may be arbitrary, it may be untidy, and it may be unfair in the view of those who get less than they would under some other alternatives. But we cannot reject the hypothesis that the recent growth in Part B spending was driven by demand, or by declines in relative user prices (both more assignment and Medigap growth) and changes in technology, both of which make beneficiaries better off. It is not that we *know* that the growth was justified, either; the proper strategy is not to base policy on an assumption that either outcome is known with certainty. Rather, proper policy faces uncertainty squarely in the face and devises arrangements that offer no guarantee of perfection after the fact, but are the best compromise with uncertainty.

In designing such policy, the most important uncertainty to recognize is the uncertainty that relative prices are a critical part of the problem. The intuitively persuasive argument from armchair economics for equalizing relative net revenues turns out to be most relevant in a perfect (but unrealistic) market economy in which no public intervention is needed. The world in which relative profitability does differ in equilibrium is a world that we know very little about—except that "reasonable" policies can produce bizarre results. Policy almost never is based on certainty, but the ambiguity here is great enough that a process of experimentation and demonstration might be wise.

The least uncertainty attaches to a proposition not about relative prices but about absolute prices. It is at least arguable that almost all Medicare prices are too high, in the limited sense that they are higher than the lowest prices needed to get doctors to supply to Medicare beneficiaries what Medicare thinks they should get. An announced policy of modest and prespecified limits on overall fee-level growth or total Part B spending may, in an analogy with Milton Friedman's advice to the Federal Reserve, be the best strategy in an uncertain world. If policy makers are bold enough to want to fine-tune in a static-filled world, they ought to specify what they want to buy and what they do not want to buy. Then prices can be designed to produce a good outcome.

## Notes

1. William Hsiao et al., *A National Study of Resource-based Relative Value Scales for Physician Services: Final Report* (Boston, Mass.: Harvard University School of Public Health, 1988).
2. R. R. Bovbjerg, P. J. Held, and M. V. Pauly, "Privatization and Bidding in the Health Care Sector," *Journal of Policy Analysis and Management*, vol. 6, no. 4 (Summer 1987), pp. 648–66.
3. Hsiao et al., *A National Study of Resource-based Relative Value Scales for Physician Services*.
4. J. M. Eisenberg, L. P. Myers, and M. V. Pauly, "How Will Changes in Physician Payment by Medicare Influence Laboratory Testing?" *Journal of the American Medical Association*, vol. 258, no. 6 (August 14, 1987), pp. 803–8.
5. See Robert G. Evans, "Supplier-Induced Demand: Some Empirical Evidence and Implications," in M. Perlman, ed., *The Economics of Health and Medical Care* (London: Macmillan, 1974), pp. 162–73; Mark V. Pauly, *Doctors and Their Workshops* (Chicago: University of Chicago Press, 1980).
6. Physician Payment Review Commission, *Annual Report to Congress*, March 1988.
7. I am indebted to John Eisenberg for suggesting this approach.
8. David Dranove, "Demand Inducement and the Physician-Patient Relationship," *Economic Inquiry*, vol. 26 (April 1988), pp. 281–98.

9. Pauly, *Doctors and Their Workshops*.
10. See Pamela Farley, "Theories of the Price and Quantity of Physician Services: A Synthesis and Critique," *Journal of Health Economics*, vol. 5 (December 1986), pp. 315–34; Jose J. Escarce, "Relative Prices for Physicians' Services," Leonard Davis Institute of Health Economics, University of Pennsylvania (December 1988, photocopied).

# Chapter 12

# The Effect of Medicare's Resource-Based Relative Value Scale on the Private Sector

In this chapter we consider the effect of the change in relative prices embodied in the Medicare resource-based relative value scale on the private sector and on commercial insurers. We use the same three behavioral models for physicians to try to predict the effects, if any, of the RBRVS on patients and insurers in the private sector. The second part of this chapter focuses on the possible responses of private insurers to Medicare's payment changes, explicitly within the framework of uncertainty about what that effect will be. Some strategies for private-sector insurers are suggested.

## RBRVS Effects Predicted by the Behavioral Models

### Profit maximization

Consider the case in which physicians are assumed to have profit maximization alone as an objective, in which profit is money income net of an implicit cost of time or wage rate. How would prices and quantities of services that physicians provide to privately insured patients change when Medicare sets some volume limits and reduces the price it pays for some services to Medicare patients? The answer depends in part on whether or not the Medicare market is assumed to be in equilibrium; that is, whether or not the volume of services in that market is limited by what patients demand, rather than by what doctors are willing to supply. (Note that the relevant demand could well be shifted upward as far as it will go by inducement. In a profit maximization model, as discussed in Chapter 3, the predictions about the qualitative effects of changes in payment do not depend on the occurrence of inducement.)

Suppose Medicare patients demand (or can be persuaded to accept) as much service as doctors are willing to supply. From the doctor's perspective, it is as if there is unlimited demand at the price Medicare sets. In contrast, for private-sector patients the physician can set his or her own price. In order to conclude that the private-sector price is not infinite, we need to ensure that the private-sector demand depends in part on what the doctor charges. Insurance coverage for a physician's service is often incomplete and carries some coinsurance. Higher physician prices often lead to higher out-of-pocket payments by privately insured patients, and these higher prices will eventually cause the patient to switch doctors or forgo the service. Uninsured patients and those whose policies carry substantial deductibles will also care about higher physician charges.

Given such a private demand curve, how does a profit-maximizing doctor decide what price to charge private-sector patients? If we assume that the quality and characteristics of services are the same in Medicare and non-Medicare markets, then the physician will determine the non-Medicare price for seeing one more private-sector patient by comparing the Medicare price with the change in total non-Medicare revenue from seeing one more such patient—that is, the marginal revenue for a private-sector, non-Medicare patient. This marginal revenue reflects the revenue obtained from selling another unit of service to non-Medicare patients. To maximize profits, the price for a service to a Medicare patient needs to be equated to the marginal revenue for a service to a non-Medicare patient, and these quantities also need to be equated to the (marginal) cost of the service. (In any situation, a firm maximizes profits by setting marginal revenue equal to marginal cost.)

It is not necessary for the non-Medicare price to equal the Medicare price. In general, the non-Medicare marginal revenue will be lower than the non-Medicare price—reflecting the price cut needed to cause the purchase of additional care—so that the non-Medicare price will be *higher*, in equilibrium, than the price Medicare sets.

To achieve a state of equilibrium the private marginal revenue must equal the Medicare price. If the Medicare price was below the private marginal revenue, "profit" could be increased by selling more non-Medicare services (which would require reducing the private price a little to increase the quantity demanded). The incentive to reduce the private price, to substitute the more profitable non-Medicare business for the Medicare business, will only go away when the same additional revenue is obtained from both types of patients.

Were Medicare to reduce the price for some service, profit maximization implies that the level of private marginal revenue would also have to be reduced, so that more output could be sold in the more profitable non-Medicare market. The conclusion, then, is that reducing the Medicare price—if it is to have any effect on private-sector patients—will lead to a *reduction* in the price charged to private customers, and a consequent increase in the volume of services they demand. If Medicare increased specific prices (e.g., for diagnosis and evaluation services), we could predict an increase in private price and a reduction in private quantity. This conclusion does, of course, depend on the assumption that there is a private market in which demand responds to price. Were that not so—were private-sector patients willing to pay any price—then profit-maximizing doctors would set infinitely high private prices. Because private prices, although high by some standards, are not infinite, one who is not willing to assume that the private market is responsive to price must then assume that physicians do not maximize profits.

This counterintuitive result, that a Medicare price cut will be fought with private price cuts, follows directly from the assumption that the physician was initially in profit-maximizing equilibrium. Raising the private price would then not be sensible, because the private price was already so high that further increases would reduce total profits. Further inducement of private demand is also not profitable, because inducement was already at its maximum. The only way left to generate the revenues to replace the less profitable Medicare business is to *lower* the private price to offer an incentive for more private patients to seek services.

Now consider the alternative case in which the amount of Medicare demand is fully satisfied at the current Medicare price. In such a case, only the amount of private services can be varied by the physician. Therefore, overall profit maximization only requires that the private price be set at the profit-maximizing level. In *this* equilibrium, seeing one more Medicare patient would add more to profit than cutting the price in order to see one more non-Medicare patient. But there is an insufficient supply of willing Medicare patients. A change in the Medicare price will then generally have *no* effect on the private price or quantity, because neither the cost nor the private demand is affected by the change in Medicare price. Although Medicare patients are made less profitable by a price cut, they are still profitable enough to cause physicians to want to treat them. A cut in the Medicare price will have an effect only if the cut is so large that Medicare patients cease to be more profitable than the marginal non-Medicare patient—and then the response will be a cut in the non-Medicare price.

These examples suggest that private insurers should have little concern about cost shifting when the Medicare price is reduced, *if* they believe that doctors are net revenue maximizers. Either there will be no effect on private-sector prices, or the prices will fall. Although the latter case would then be expected to involve an increase in volume for persons who have coverage with coinsurance (because a fall in total price leads to a fall in the amount of cost sharing), total quantity for the market as a whole will probably increase less than proportionately, because market demand is not very responsive to price. In such cases, the total cost of benefits to private insurers will fall.

Of course, if doctors were ordered to match Medicare price cuts with price cuts to their private patients, then private payers would pay less than if there were no such order. But this difference does not reflect the elimination of cost shifting; it merely describes the consequences of the imposition of the rule.

### Target income or inducement

This generally benign result on the private sector could be sharply reversed if the relevant model of physician behavior involves demand inducement constrained by the physician's utility function—the target-income approach. Price changes caused by the RBRVS may affect inducement if the willingness to induce for one service is related to the amount of inducement for other services. For example, if the initial equilibrium was one in which the additional net income per unit of distasteful inducement "effort" was equalized across all services, the most direct effect of a price change will be to upset this equality. This will also lead to more inducement for private-sector services with unchanged prices. The notion is that, because inducement of now lower-priced Medicare services has become less profitable, the inducement effort will be shifted to other relatively more profitable services—both to Medicare services experiencing price increases and, unfortunately, to all non-Medicare services.

If, for example, the price of surgery for Medicare patients is reduced, we might expect to see some inducement by surgeons for both surgical and nonsurgical services to non-Medicare patients. There is no reason why there should be a simple surgery-for-surgery offset; the inducement effect would be expected to be felt across the board, and could well be greater for nonsurgical services such as diagnostic tests or even surgeon office visits. Moreover, how large this effect will be is not known.

It is also possible, as noted earlier, that a price cut for a set of Medicare services will cause an increase in the quantity of those services, if the price-reduced services form a large enough share of a physician's total income. A sufficiently large decline in income may increase the willingness of a doctor to induce demand for all services he or she provides, including those that undergo a price cut. But this perverse effect for Medicare should offer no consolation to non-Medicare patients or their insurers, because a positive effect on quantity for a service with a lowered price only implies an even larger positive effect on volume for all other services rendered by the physicians experiencing large price declines. That is, even if a cut in Medicare surgical fees leads to an increase in surgery for Medicare patients, it can also lead to an increase in the volume of all services—surgical and nonsurgical—that surgeons provide to non-Medicare patients.

The reverse holds true for services whose Medicare prices are increased. An increase in price would prompt more inducement of that service and, in itself, less inducement of all other services that the same physicians provide. Likewise, an increase in total income from Medicare business for particular physicians would prompt them to reduce the amount of inducement they undertake from non-Medicare business.

### Patient agency

The physician who is a perfect agent for his or her patients may change the quantity of Medicare services as changes in out-of-pocket cost sharing prompt patients to desire more of the now cheaper services and fewer of the now more costly services. The perfect agent for non-Medicare patients should not change behavior at all, however, because there is no direct change in either the cost or the benefit from those services.

## Evidence from the Medicaid Program

Medicare has traditionally tried to tie its prices to what the private sector charges, although the limitation on the rate of increase embedded in the Medicare economic index has caused Medicare payment rates to fall behind those in the private sector. Likewise, Medicare has traditionally allowed balance billing (within some limits), but has offered some incentives to accept the Medicare payment rate as payment in full. In contrast, the Medicaid program has aggressively lowered what it pays to well below the price charged to private-sector patients, and has forbidden doctors to bill for the balance. Because it appears that Medicare may be moving in both of these directions, what lessons does Medicaid offer? Probably the most convincing lesson from Medicaid is that, in the aggregate, reducing prices reduces the willingness of doctors to accept Medicaid patients. To be sure, Medicaid prices are low, and Medicaid patients frequently do not have access to individual doctors. Nevertheless, it appears that for those practices not dominated by Medicare business, services rendered to Medicare patients will likewise decline if Medicare cuts its fees to the same extent as Medicaid has done.

## Strategies for Private Insurers

Given the uncertainty about the response of physicians to Medicare's reimbursement and price changes and limits, what are sensible strategies for private-sector payers? One watershed decision a payer must make is whether or not it wishes to use the occasion of the "Medicaidization" of Medicare to increase the access, quality, and attractiveness of physician services covered under its plan. Even if premiums must rise to cover costs, judicious choice of a marketing strategy could offer the prospect of even higher buyer willingness to pay. This would seem to be a sensible strategy for insurance plans marketed to higher-income buyers and firms, ones to whom quality, the absence of delay and hassle, and the ability to get the doctor one wants are all characteristics of high value.

We suspect that the majority of private-sector buyers will not be so willing to pay higher premiums, however, given the current high level of pressure for cost containment in the private sector. If an insurer has a relatively small market share, so that it cannot, itself, force down the prices doctors charge, what can it do? We offer four potential strategies for individual payers—matching price changes, managing balance billing, establishing a preferred provider network, and monitoring volume—as well as one for the industry as a whole—organizing collective action.

### Matching price changes

Consider the stylized Medicare payment policy in which Medicare payment for some surgical procedure is reduced and Medicare payment for office visits is increased. What should a private insurer with a relatively small market share do in response?

One might suppose, first of all, that the insurer would need to increase what it pays for office visits; otherwise, physicians will refuse to provide visits to non-Medicare beneficiaries. For this to happen among physicians generally, however, doctors would have to increase the quantity of office visits that Medicare patients demand. It seems plausible that, before the price change, the volume of Medicare visits was constrained by demand. There are not many Medicare beneficiaries who seek visits and are refused. The copayment for Medicare office visits will rise when the reimbursement level for visits increases, so that increasing the quantity of such visits will require that there be either inducement of the demand for visits or an increase in the "quality" or style of a visit.

In the latter case, Medicare visits become more costly and therefore less profitable, so that there is no need for the private payer to pay more if it chooses to buy "lower-quality" visits. In the former case, private payers presumably would not want to promote inducement of visits for their enrollees. The only real need for raising the private price would be if there was strong inducement of demand for Medicare visits. If Medicare inducement is limited in extent, physicians would still be willing to see private-sector patients for less than Medicare pays. Private-sector visits would be relatively less profitable than Medicare visits, but they would still show positive profits—and there would be no profitable Medicare patients queuing up to be seen.

What about the surgery or other procedure subjected to a Medicare price cut? In a world in which there is little inducement, physicians might be willing to accept similarly lower fees for these services for their private-sector patients, if the private insurer is able to offer a credible threat to send those patients elsewhere should the surgeon refuse the lower price. A single patient seeking care probably does not pose such a threat, but even an insurer with modest volume might at least match some part of Medicare's price cuts. Saying anything more than this is difficult in the absence of information about voluntary discriminatory pricing by physicians. Strategic questions (e.g., if I match the Medicare price cuts for your enrollees, will all my patients know about it and seek the same cuts?) are likely to be important in the short run.

We suspect that, were prevailing prices for surgery indeed excessive before Medicare instituted its cuts, there would eventually be erosion of the prices for surgery charged to all payers, but the pattern might be uneven and slow. As is usual in such cases, the insurer who can promise to deliver substantial volume in exchange for a price cut that resembles Medicare's, or who can threaten to take away substantial volume if a cut is refused, is likely to be able to extract concessions.

Eagerness to match Medicare price cuts and reluctance to match Medicare price increases would seem to describe the best posture for a private insurer. Obtaining control over a noticeable block of volume—the share probably does not need to be nearly as large as Medicare's—will help. But matching lower prices may nevertheless prove difficult. Medicaid fee levels, as well as some Medicare fees, have been below private fees in some areas of the country for some time, and yet the differential remains. Private insurers have not been able to match the already lower Medicare fees in these circumstances thus far, so they may not be able to do so to any greater extent under the new fees.

The main threat to private-insurer costs comes from the possibility of spillover inducement. This threat is far from certain, but keeping one's own prices from getting too high relative to Medicare's is a good

protection strategy when it is feasible. The other strategy is to redou-
ble utilization review efforts applied to procedures in which Medicare
margins are lower than private margins.

## Managing balance billing

If the payer does reduce reimbursement levels to correspond to what
Medicare has done, its insured population may be subject to higher
balance billing. That is, the physician whose reimbursement for a visit
is reduced may increase what he or she charges the patient. Medicare
has placed limits on such balance billing. But can, or should, private
insurers do so? A possible strategy is to make the existence of balance
billing, its rationale, and its use by particular physicians a much more
explicit object of marketing strategy. To see the rationale for this strategy,
one should first note that there are two reasons for balance billing, one
negative and one positive. The negative reason is, of course, that high
prices charged by doctors may represent use of monopoly power, usually
based on the relatively greater ignorance of the buyer about the quality
of the service to be provided and the prices charged by other doctors.
To be sure, additional balance billing in response to a reimbursement cut
may represent exercise of monopoly power that previously had not been
used by the doctor. There is, however, another reason for balance billing.
It may represent the higher price needed to induce the doctor to supply
as much service, in a quantitative or qualitative sense, as buyers want.
The doctor with the best skills or the best reputation in town may well
find that people seek to use more of those services than the doctor is
willing to supply. The solution, then, is to raise the price charged. Doing
so will induce the doctor to supply more and induce buyers to use other
doctors and thus demand less. In effect, the balance-billed amount, if paid
willingly by a buyer, represents mutually agreed upon compensation for
better services, whereas potentially great harm is done by prohibiting
such voluntary exchanges.

The problem is to distinguish between appropriate and inappropriate balance billing. Because lack of consumer information is at the root
of inappropriate balance billing, one strategy private payers may find
worthwhile is to try to highlight the aspects of price and quality that are
in question. Specifically, providing information on doctors who do not
balance bill, and on the access and quality of those who do, may help
consumers to feel more comfortable with the existence of balance billing.
A designated list of high-quality doctors who agree not to balance bill,
along with a list of doctors who do balance bill because of evidence of
higher quality or higher demand, should enable consumers to choose.
This assumes we can measure the quality of an individual doctor's

outcomes, at least well enough to permit reasonable choices. Those who do not want to pay more will be able to find a set of providers who satisfy their desires, whereas those who do desire (and are willing to pay for) additional quality will have access to an information-based list that will tell them who does what for how much. They can then make their own choices, in a reasonably well-informed way.

For most private insurers other than Blue Cross and Blue Shield, the market power needed to enforce limits on balance billing will be lacking. Such limits therefore will be ineffective in dealing directly with inappropriate balance billing.

## A preferred provider network

It would also be possible for an insurer to carry the strategy of identifying doctors who agree to accept a lower price as payment in full one step further, toward a true preferred provider organization or PPO. Those providers who agree to accept some price as payment in full can be so designated, and financial incentives can be built into a reimbursement plan to encourage patients to use them. The incentives usually take the form of higher out-of-pocket payments, perhaps even in excess of the balance-billed amount, if those who are insured use nonpreferred providers.

## Volume monitoring

Some private-sector insurers are, at least nominally, shielded from physicians' pricing reactions to changes in Medicare payments, because insurers reimburse up to a fixed dollar amount per unit of service. They need not raise the benefits they pay out just because prices have risen. (Of course, if reimbursement levels are tied to the distribution of actual prices, there will be a link. But there is no necessary reason why this link needs to be preserved.) Insurers are vulnerable, however, to adjustments in volume that may ensue. As indicated above, the likelihood and the magnitude of those adjustments are very difficult to estimate; there is a good chance that, at least for some services in some markets, there will be no increases or decreases in private-sector volumes when Medicare reimbursements rise. Given this rampant uncertainty, a sensible strategy for private insurers would be to monitor carefully for Medicare-induced volume changes, and take action only if those changes occur in large enough magnitude to require it.

Monitoring volume change is not, in itself, a simple task. Some index or indicator of total volume must be constructed, data must be accumulated on a timely basis, and—most challenging of all—effects on volume caused by Medicare pricing polices must be separated from other effects on volume. At a minimum, a baseline trend must be established, and effects of changing demographics or changing technology must be separated out. Here, as elsewhere, the degree of precision sought depends on the usefulness of the information. However, particularly if drastic steps are contemplated to deal with the threat of volume changes, there should be substantial confidence that the event has in fact taken place.

## Organizing collective or coordinated action

Individual commercial insurers lack the market power needed to force prices down or to force physicians to accept limits on balance billing. It will require government sanctions—at a minimum, waiver of antitrust laws, and probably also state-enforced power to punish insurers or physicians who renege on the agreement—to allow a collective attempt to match Medicare pricing *and* limits on balance billing. Only Blue Cross and Blue Shield has a chance to match Medicare without such waivers, and state sanctions will probably still be required. Should such efforts to achieve collective buyer market power ("monopsony," in economic jargon) be sought by private insurers?

Such attempts should be approached with extreme caution. It is by no means obvious that, in the long run, such actions will enhance insurer profit or the ability to break even. Insurance is a financial device for transferring and spreading risks, and it can work as well with high benefit payments, caused by high prices, as with those caused by low prices. Of course, after premiums are set and collected, reducing payouts by reducing provider prices will raise profits; conversely, unexpected price increases will cause losses. Once insurers anticipate the provider price changes, however, a lower level of prices will, in the high competitive insurance market, lead to lower premiums, not higher profits. The gain from lower prices ultimately goes to consumers who pay less for insurance, not to insurers who profit more.

Would consumer welfare and overall welfare be increased by changes in relative or absolute provider prices? Lower prices can lower insurance premiums, but they also can lower access (quantity supplied) and quality. Much of the discussion in this book has been directed at that question, and we have come up with a nihilistic answer. No one knows, and the effect could be as negative as it is positive for some or all consumers. What we can say is that, if the price is pushed low enough, an effective aggregate price reduction will produce some eventual reduction in supply. In addition, forcing down provider prices simply redistributes real income from providers to consumers. That is, a price-control strategy may increase consumer welfare only by reducing physician welfare. If we knew that physicians currently receive an unjustly high level of income, we might (at least those of us who are not physicians) feel more confident in recommending such a redistribution (based on a theory of distributive justice), even though there is no warrant for it in economic theory. If we knew that doctors' incomes are currently inflated by monopoly power, we might feel more confident in recommending price cuts, although a better solution would be to remove or weaken the source of the monopoly power. Because so much is uncertain, however, none of these recommendations can be made with great confidence.

What is certain is that if physician price setting is brought under the power of government, politics will intervene. In theory, this is not necessarily bad, although in practice Americans have been justifiably skeptical of the ability of government to make matters better in circumstances in which government intervention is not obviously necessary. We cannot offer counsel on practical politics here. We can only offer a strong word of caution, especially to a private industry that (we assume) would prefer to remain private.

Evidence may eventually indicate that collective action is needed. Current evidence is not sufficient. Here again, waiting to see what will happen, monitoring carefully so that we know what is happening, and having institutional mechanisms (such as the Physician Payment Review Commission) in place to take action if needed are all part of the best of current strategies.

## Should Private Insurers Try Other Devices to Control Physician Volume?

Even had Medicare not adopted RBRVS, private insurers would still be interested in trying to limit or control the volume of physician services. Of the devices we have reviewed, which are the best ones for them to use?

The major difference between Medicare and commercial (non–Blue Cross) private insurers is that the latter have a much smaller share of total volumes. Although this gives private insurers less leverage, it does allow them more flexibility. In particular, they can experiment with alternative devices, and they can use the market test—what do buyers want?—to select among the devices. An important message for private insurers, then, is to continue to use this flexibility and not to copy the public system in every detail. Even with regard to physician reimbursement levels, some insurers may want to copy Medicare while others may choose to go in exactly the opposite direction. For utilization review, for copayments, and for the other devices, the same message regarding the value of experimentation applies.

With utilization review, for example, private insurers can be much more aggressive than Medicare because private insurers are not hobbled by political pressure to the extent that Medicare is. Moreover, private insurers can reasonably argue that an aggressive UR policy, even if it seriously inconveniences the insured, rewards them in turn with lower premiums. (Medicare, in contrast, gives three-fourths of any reward from harassing the elderly and their physicians to general federal revenues and uses at most one-fourth to lower Part B premiums.) This suggests that designing aggressive utilization review, publicizing its potential for cost savings, and offering it on the market may be a desirable strategy for private insurers.

On the cost sharing or copayment issue, it is fair to say that higher copayments would reduce the level of cost and use, but they would be resisted because they cause reductions in the level of protection against risk. Here again, some insurance purchasers may be willing to tolerate such an increase if they are serious about holding down health insurance costs. Sometimes cost-sharing strategies are rejected, especially in labor-management negotiations, in favor of managed care arrangements that try to preserve generous coverage and promise to control costs as well. It is too soon to say whether these arrangements will work, but it is reasonable to suppose that they will not always work, whereas cost sharing is much more consistent in its effect. Some type of repackaging of cost sharing, perhaps as a no-claims bonus, might be a sensible strategy.

The evidence reviewed here does not support the view that there is a single, flawless method for controlling the volume of physician services. Our overall conclusion is that experimentation and monitoring are the best strategies for the private sector.

# Current Approaches to Controlling Volume and Intensity: Results of Two Surveys

## The Surveys

We conducted two surveys to assess the range of approaches that all Medicare Part B carriers and a sample of private health insurance carriers use to control volume and intensity. The first survey, designed by the University of Minnesota's Division of Health Services Research and Policy in consultation with the Bureau of Program Operations (BPO) of the Health Care Financing Administration (HCFA), was a poll of Medicare Part B carriers. Its purpose was to analyze the effectiveness of methods for ensuring that Medicare payments are made only for medically necessary physicians' services. The second survey, designed by the Health Insurance Association of America (HIAA) with advice from the University of Minnesota, polled private insurance carriers on their methods to control the volume and intensity of physician services. Each of these carriers was asked about its commercial and group health insurance business in three areas: commercial insurance products, PPOs, and HMOs.

The survey of Medicare carriers was mailed on 12 September 1988 to 46 carriers. A cover letter from HCFA's Director of the Office of Program Operations Procedures urged carriers to cooperate with the survey. Two weeks later the University of Minnesota followed up with a telephone call to each recipient to review any problem areas and write down the answers to the survey questions. Carriers were then instructed to return the survey by mail. This method of using mail surveys and telephone follow-up has been found to be an accurate method for collecting complex information such as that requested by the carrier survey. By early November, 96 percent (44) of the surveys had been returned.

The HIAA survey was conducted in June and July of 1988 by trained telephone interviewers from HIAA's office in Washington, DC. One hundred twenty-three companies were selected from a sampling universe of 194 companies; 100 percent responded.

Both surveys contained closed- and open-ended questions regarding carriers' programs to control volume and intensity. In closed-ended questions, the respondent was presented with a limited number of categories from which to select an answer, or was asked for a numerical or qualitative rating of the effectiveness of a volume and intensity control. In open-ended questions, the respondent was offered more latitude in his or her answer (e.g., What is your overall feeling toward the effectiveness of a control?). Although open-ended questions are often useful for understanding the context of the topic being studied, it may be difficult to categorize and compare responses to such questions.

In reporting the results of these surveys, we focus first on Medicare carriers and then on private carriers. Private carriers are divided into two groups—conventional group and individual insurance businesses, and PPOs—for which results are reported separately.

## Results: Medicare Carriers

Medical review screens are manual or automated edits designed to suspend the processing of services that meet specified selection criteria. Services are then evaluated to determine their medical necessity. In general, medical review screens may be of two types: prepayment and postpayment. These screens are distinguished by whether selection and review occurs before or after a claim has been paid.

### Prepayment review activities

Until recently there was only one mandated prepayment screen: claims from physicians who made multiple visits to nursing home patients were automatically reviewed. Thirteen national screens, all dealing with the volume and intensity of physicians' services, are now mandated by HCFA. Claims that exceed certain limits or guidelines (e.g., more than 31 hospital visits per three-month period) are reviewed for medical necessity before they are paid. The carrier (typically using a nurse, physician, or clerk) reviews the claims against criteria of medical necessity. Claims deemed unnecessary may be denied or reduced. Carriers may set tighter guidelines for screening than those mandated by HCFA, and there are numerous local screens in addition to the 13 nationally mandated screens.

Table A.1 shows how many carriers who responded to our survey had implemented the screen before the mandated date and how many were using a screening index tighter than the mandated one. Although many carriers had implemented the screens before they were mandated, few were using tighter screening measures. One explanation for why carriers do not exceed the mandated guidelines is ignorance. We discovered that for most of the screens implemented prior to the mandated date, tighter measures were relaxed to conform with the federal mandate because carriers apparently thought that HCFA would not allow tighter restrictions. For example, although eight carriers were using screening measures tighter than the federal mandate for chiropractic services, on close examination it became apparent that most of them prohibited more than 12 spinal manipulations per year, or one per month (the mandated guideline). An extra screen catches suppliers who perform six spinal manipulations within three months. Two carriers implemented very strict screens: one reviewed all chiropractic claims for medical necessity, and one required radiographs or x-rays to substantiate the claims.

Carriers were asked to describe any problems they encountered in implementing mandated prepayment screens. Responses to this open-ended question indicated a general increase in physician complaints about government interference in medical practice but no significant problems. Several carriers offered constructive suggestions about how to implement a new screen. They suggested that it should be publicized in advance (e.g., through newsletters). One noted that the implementation date was effective immediately and gave little time to instruct the providers on the new screens. Once the provider was notified and edits or audits were in place, no major problems were encountered. Interestingly, most complaints about screens came from podiatrists and chiropractors. One carrier commented that "chiropractors are very organized and they continually ask for further reviews."

Asked to identify the skill level of the person who normally performed medical review for mandated screens, 27 carriers reported using a claims examiner with limited medical training, 12 used nurses, and 5 used physicians. Although not required to do so, many carriers also mentioned a second skill level; for most, the person at this level was a nurse.

Carriers were given the opportunity to "sound off" by naming up to three mandated screens that in their opinion were not cost-effective. Only six carriers failed to name at least one ineffective screen. The number of times each mandated screen was cited as ineffective is shown in Table A.2. Several features are noteworthy. First, carriers consistently rated certain screens as ineffective. Routine foot care and injections topped this

**Table A.1**　Information on Nationally Mandated Prepayment Screens

| Screen | Mandated Date (month/year) | Number of Carriers Who Had Prior Implementation (out of 44) | Mandated Measure | Number of Carriers Who Had Tighter Measures (out of 44) |
|---|---|---|---|---|
| Routine foot care | 10/84 | 6 | 1 treatment per 60 days | 3 |
| Mycotic nails | 10/84 | 11 | 1 treatment per 60 days | 2 |
| Nursing home visits | 10/84 | 16 | 1 visit per month | 1 |
| New patient office visits | 10/84 | 7 | 1 comprehensive physical exam per carrier history period | 3 |
| Holter and real-time monitoring | 10/84 | 6 | 1 instance per 6 months | 0 |
| Chiropractic | 1/86 | 32 | 12 spinal manipulations per year | 8 |
| Concurrent care | 1/86 | 34 | 1 doctor of same specialty billing for inhospital services on same day | 3 |
| Hospital visits | 1/86 | 29 | 31 times in 3 months | 5 |
| Comprehensive office visits | 1/86 | 28 | 1 per 6 months | 2 |
| Skilled nursing facility (SNF) visits | 1/86 | 33 | 2 subsequent care visits in first week, 1 visit per week thereafter | 6 |
| Injections | 1/86 | 30 | 24 per year | 4 |
| Urological supplies | 1/86 | 28 | 2 catheters per month | 1 |
| Replacement of postcataract external prosthetic contact lens | 1/86 | 27* | 1 per eye per year | 2 |

*2 missing values.

list, followed by urological supplies and postcataract contact lenses. In response to another question, carriers noted that they had observed that the foot care screen was difficult to implement. Second, only four carriers viewed chiropractic prepayment screening as ineffective, although this was the screen most likely to have implementation problems. Finally, almost all rated the following screens as cost-effective: nursing home visits, new patient office visits, concurrent care, and comprehensive office visits.

We noted previously that carriers used numerous local screens in addition to the 13 mandated ones. We asked each carrier how many such screens it used. The median response was 21; one carrier had 121 local screens. Apparently carriers are quite active in this area. Each was asked to recommend up to three of these screens to include in the list of nationally mandated screens. Although responses were extremely varied, several regular patterns appeared. First, many carriers believed that consultations were being abused. This was mentioned about 20 times. Second, and closely following concerns over abuse of consultations, was

**Table A.2** Carriers' Opinions about Ineffective Mandated Screens

| | Number of Times Mentioned | | | |
|---|---|---|---|---|
| *Screen* | *1 Mention* | *2 Mentions* | *3 Mentions* | *Total* |
| Routine foot care | 11 | 4 | 1 | 16 |
| Mycotic nails | 0 | 3 | 2 | 5 |
| Nursing home visits | 3 | 0 | 0 | 3 |
| New patient office visits | 0 | 1 | 0 | 1 |
| Holter and real-time monitoring | 0 | 1 | 3 | 4 |
| Chiropractic | 0 | 1 | 3 | 4 |
| Concurrent care | 0 | 0 | 1 | 1 |
| Hospital visits | 6 | 1 | 1 | 8 |
| Comprehensive office visits | 1 | 2 | 0 | 3 |
| Skilled nursing facility (SNF) visits | 2 | 1 | 2 | 5 |
| Injections | 12 | 4 | 3 | 19 |
| Urological supplies | 1 | 7 | 2 | 10 |
| Replacement of postcataract external prosthetic contact lens | 2 | 7 | 3 | 12 |
| No screens thought to be ineffective | 6 | 12 | 23 | 41 |

concern both about the number of hospital visits per hospitalization and about the number of visits per time period. Third, carriers recommended screening office visits more carefully than was mandated by Medicare. Finally, hospital emergency room visits were cited as an area to review.

Also of interest are the services or procedures that carriers did not think were subject to inappropriate billing and that, therefore, did not need national screens. These included multichannel lab studies, vascular studies and venipuncture, critical care, seat lifts, and ambulance services.

## Postpayment review activities

Postpayment medical review is a process by which practice patterns of physicians or suppliers are compared to statistical norms for them and their specialty groups. The purpose of this process is to identify suppliers whose practice patterns depart from recognized norms, and to correct overutilization of services by recovery of overpayments and education.

Knowledge of service area data is one of the most important requirements in operating a postpayment screen. Carriers therefore are directed to "use acceptable statistical techniques in [their] postpayment utilization safeguard system to array data by specialty group." Once the data have been analyzed, carriers are directed to "use the appropriate statistical tools which will best identify the physician/supplier who needs further investigation by the postpayment medical review (MR) staff."[1]

Carriers are required to make postpayment pattern-of-practice comparisons for the following service categories: office visits, home visits, hospital visits, skilled nursing facility (SNF) visits, injections, EKGs, surgery, office lab services, office diagnostic x-ray, and physical therapy. There are two peer practice pattern comparison ratios to calculate for each service: Ratio I is the number of services provided by a physician or supplier per 100 beneficiaries; Ratio II is the number of services per beneficiary who actually received services in that category. After calculating these ratios, carriers are instructed to determine the point at which the ratio exceeds the norm. They may use percentiles, index values, medians, modes, and so forth.

In the carrier survey, we asked each Medicare Part B carrier to furnish the critical value of Ratios I and II that would cause a supplier to be selected for postpayment review. The carriers responded that critical values could not be determined by simple formulas. Instead, more complex methods were used. These typically involved selecting a point on the distribution of ratios. In 14 cases the point selected was two standard deviations above the mean. Three carriers used a standard deviation other than 2.0, and two used 2.0 standard deviations plus the top 150 physicians.

Three carriers automatically reviewed the top physicians within each category, whether or not these physicians had unusual practice patterns. The chosen cutoffs varied widely: 20, 200, and 300 physicians were selected for review by various carriers. Four carriers used percentile cutoffs, reviewing the top 25, 20, 5, and 3 percent of all physicians. Seven carriers used a specified percentage above the mean to select physicians for review. Both these methods are similar to using a standard deviation–based cutoff, although this standard deviation would vary widely (for example, reviewing the top 5 percent of all physicians is similar to using a 1.65 standard deviation cutoff, but reviewing the top 25 percent is similar to using a much lower cutoff—about two-thirds of a standard deviation above the mean). Six carriers had no specific standards for postpayment review, two did not answer the question, one gave an answer that could not be classified, and only two used a specified number for each ratio.

It appears, consequently, that carriers use widely different postpayment standards. Although these differences may reflect optimal adaptations to local environments, it is also possible that some standards lack a carefully justified basis. This is especially likely for those that are based on reviewing a predetermined number of physicians. Unless the system is based on an implicit recognition that these physicians have unusual practice patterns, it is difficult to argue that a simple numerical formula (e.g., reviewing the top 20 physicians) is a well-designed postpayment medical review strategy.

As in the case of prepayment review, each carrier was asked to name the skill level of the person who normally performed postpayment medical review. Nurses were mentioned 24 times, followed by 12 mentions of claims examiners with limited medical training. These responses clearly indicate that postpayment MR is a more highly skilled function than prepayment review. Fourteen carriers mentioned a second person who performed postpayment MR, usually a physician or nurse.

## Use of collapsed procedure codes

Collapsed coding may be a desirable method for controlling volume and expenditures, although our theoretical discussion indicates that the effect of coding changes may be ambiguous. In practice, how many Medicare carriers have implemented coding system changes, and what is the opinion of those who have implemented them regarding their effectiveness? Each carrier was asked if it had changed the coding of physician services to prevent physicians from "upcoding" procedures (e.g., Has the carrier reduced the number of office visit codes it recognizes for payment purposes?).

To our surprise, carriers placed a different interpretation on this seemingly straightforward question. Many responded that they had implemented coding system changes, but what they described was actually a "downcoding" screen. For example, if a physician submitted two claims for initial office visits from the same patient, the second claim was automatically downgraded to a code for a follow-up visit. When the interviewer attempted to clarify this question, carriers responded that they were required by law to recognize HCPCS codes (i.e., the procedure codes used in the Medicare program) on the claims. Their interpretation of this requirement was that HCPCS codes must also be recognized for billing. It did not occur to them that two codes could be combined or collapsed for billing (e.g., that initial and follow-up office visits could be paid at a single blended rate).

Only one carrier appeared to have a coding system program that went beyond the downgrading screen. This carrier described its unique approach as follows:

> Although codes were not changed to prevent upcoding, many of the allowances are the same. This occurred when we converted to HCPCS with pricing being equal for many levels contained in CPT-4. Therefore, upcoding is somewhat controlled by the pricing and payments.

Unfortunately, this carrier had not formally evaluated the effectiveness of its coding program. Thus, no evidence is available by which to judge the effect of the coding changes on cost or utilization.

### Use of service bundling

Next, carriers were asked if they extensively "bundled" physician services into broader categories (e.g., global fees for surgery). Most carriers have such programs for surgery. One carrier remarked sarcastically that global fees for surgery had been used "since the beginning of time" by carriers in that state. Carriers applied global surgical fees in different ways, some of which were extremely creative. One carrier's approach was described as follows:

> ...policy calls for bundling of ancillary services as well as pre- and postoperative care. There are approximately 700 ancillary combinations. One of our most common combinations is physical therapy treatment to one area plus two or more modalities (e.g., whirlpool, paraffin bath). . . .

Another carrier achieved global surgical fees by automatically denying pre- and postoperative visits, diagnostics, and incidental surgical procedures.

Despite their use of global fees for surgery, few carriers extended the bundling concept to other services. Responses to an open-ended question revealed these exceptions: three carriers had a single fee for automated lab panels; and two carriers applied bundling to all bills for the same month, place of service, type of service, procedure code, and provider number (except for pathology, anesthesiology, and psychiatric services that have specific bundling guidelines).

## Other volume controls

The last question on the carrier survey gave respondents the opportunity to describe other techniques for controlling volume and intensity that they had used successfully under Part B of Medicare. Responses to this open-ended question were read and analyzed. The most frequently mentioned activity was physician education. This often took the form of simple newsletters. More comprehensive educational programs involved the carrier's provider relations department in telephone contacts or on-site visits to the doctors. Although the effectiveness of educational programs is difficult to evaluate, several carriers mentioned high rates of physician compliance, and one even cited a "savings" of almost $1 million.

It appears that education is most effective if conducted in a nonadversarial fashion. One carrier described the following approach:

> The PR (provider relations) department presents monthly seminars to educate providers/suppliers. Quarterly bulletins are sent. We have the ability to print messages at the bottom of EOMBs (explanation of medical benefits). The postpayment unit presents documentation seminars at hospitals and for physician groups. We work closely with our Medical Director to keep abreast of the current patterns in medical practice. Physicians/suppliers who present patterns of overutilization can be put on a prepayment review to better control his [sic] volume of work processed and collect data to educate him.

Similar comments could be made about the educational programs that other carriers used. This nonadversarial approach supports our analysis of clinical guidelines and professional education and the finding that guidelines and education are more likely to be effective when they are clearly defined, data based, professionally derived, and drawn from respected sources.

Another general conclusion to be drawn from these open-ended responses is that carriers know who the "bad doctors" are. Several mentioned that postpayment review identified individual physicians who showed patterns of upgrading codes and overutilization. Specific screens may be devised for these providers. For example, one carrier automatically denied specified procedures when billed by a designated physician. Another noted that postpayment review identified several physicians who showed patterns of upgrading. Prepayment screens, which were developed for these physicians, reduce the level of payment, if documentation for the higher code was not provided. Finally, the carriers claimed to have aggressive fraud and abuse programs for physicians who habitually abuse the Medicare program.

## Results: Private Carriers

The Health Insurance Association of America's Managed Care Survey was conducted under subcontract in the summer of 1988 as part of our larger HCFA study of physician volume. HIAA represents 194 dues-paying organizations that write 85 percent of the commercial health insurance sold in the United States. The objective of the survey was to document the mechanisms that commercial insurers use to control the rising cost of health care services. Because HIAA researchers had conducted a similar survey during the summer of 1986, it was possible to document changes in cost-control efforts during the intervening two years, as well as to take a snapshot of current practices.

### Methods

In the spring of 1988, HIAA researchers sent a letter to the executive responsible for the group, individual, preferred provider organization, and health maintenance organization lines of business. The letter described the survey, listed specific questions, and indicated that a HIAA researcher would be calling shortly.

The sample included 123 of the 194 dues-paying organizations. The sampling frame was stratified according to prior information about the lines of business each insurer had entered. All insurers known to have entered the HMO and PPO markets were surveyed. Survey results are presented in two formats. One approach shows what a typical insurer is doing. Here, the unit of observation is the individual insurer—the number of respondents to the HIAA survey is weighted to equal the number of insurers in the dues-paying universe. The second format presents developments for the commercial insurance industry as a whole. In this case, each insurer is weighted by its relevant volume of business. Thus, large insurers count considerably more than small insurers in this presentation.

HIAA researchers interviewed a maximum of four executives with each insurer (group, individual, PPO, and HMO executives). The typical interview lasted 15 to 25 minutes. As stated earlier, 100 percent of the interviews were successfully completed. Item response rates exceeded 90 percent for most questions.

## Conventional group and individual insurance

Group and individual insurers reimburse physicians largely on the basis of usual, customary, and reasonable (UCR) charges. Figures A.1 and A.2 (both based on percentage of business) show that UCR covers 74 percent of conventional group insurance business and 56 percent of individual business. For group insurers there has been a slight movement toward billed charges (that is, paying the full billed amount) during the past two years.

When the company was the unit of observation, HIAA found that 111 of 132 group insurers used UCR. The next most popular reimbursement method, used by 12 companies, was billed charges. Only six insurers used "controlled" methods (discounted charges, fee schedule, or capitation) and three used "other" methods of paying physicians.

### *Utilization review activities*

Utilization review (UR) is clearly the most popular technique to control hospital utilization in conventional health insurance. Most companies offer more than one type of UR in their group business. For example, 120 companies provide preadmission certification, 109 provide concurrent review, and 85 provide retrospective review of inpatient care in their group business.

Utilization review grew at a rapid pace between 1986 and 1988 in group business. By 1988, 45 percent of group business was covered by preadmission certification, and slightly more was subjected to concurrent and retrospective review (Figure A.3). However, UR focuses on keeping patients out of hospitals rather than controlling inappropriate care in ambulatory settings. Only 9 percent of group business uses physician profiles (Figure A.3). The individual business market is now at the "take-off" stage with regard to utilization review (Figure A.4).

Of the 69 companies that had formally evaluated the effectiveness of preadmission certification, 56 believed that it reduces the total cost of group insurance. Only one company reported an increase in total cost; the others were either undecided or responded "don't know" to the survey. The average decrease in total cost was estimated by 52 companies to be 7 percent. Companies that had not formally evaluated their preadmission certification were asked about their overall feeling toward the technique's effectiveness. The most popular response was "somewhat

**Figure A.1**  How Did Conventional Insurers Pay Physicians for Their Services in 1986 and 1988?

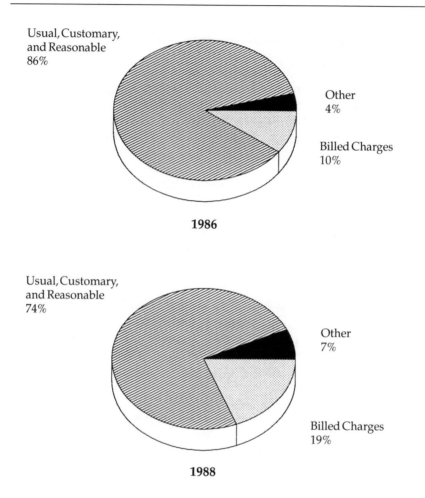

Usual, Customary, and Reasonable 86%

Other 4%

Billed Charges 10%

**1986**

Usual, Customary, and Reasonable 74%

Other 7%

Billed Charges 19%

**1988**

*Sources:* HIAA Managed Care Surveys, 1986 and 1988.

effective," although some companies believed that the program was effective only after it was implemented, and that its effectiveness was di- minished over time. Similar opinions were voiced about the effectiveness of concurrent review. Only one company had a negative opinion of its concurrent review program, based on a formal evaluation. Retrospective

**Figure A.2**  How Did Insurers Pay Hospitals and Doctors under Individual Policies in 1988?

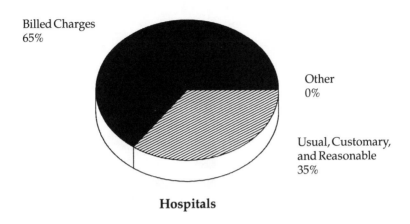

Billed Charges
65%

Other
0%

Usual, Customary,
and Reasonable
35%

**Hospitals**

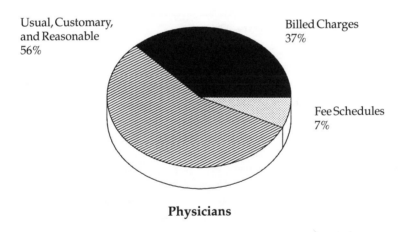

Usual, Customary,
and Reasonable
56%

Billed Charges
37%

Fee Schedules
7%

**Physicians**

*Source:* HIAA Managed Care Survey, 1988.

review, the activity least likely to be evaluated, had a mixed reception from the insurers. Figure A.5 summarizes insurers' perceptions regarding the effectiveness of utilization management in controlling claims costs in their group business. Individual insurers were more enthusiastic about UR (Figure A.6).

**Figure A.3**    Percentage of Group Business Covered by Various
Utilization Management Programs, 1988

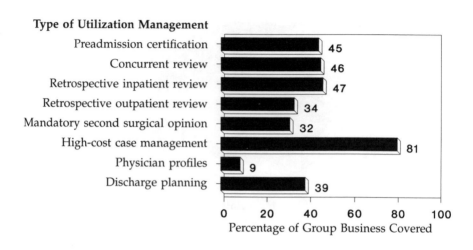

*Source:* HIAA Managed Care Survey, 1988.

Although companies agreed that UR reduced total cost, they gave it poor marks for controlling cost and utilization outside the hospital. Most respondents who answered this question believed that preadmission certification increased cost and utilization outside the hospital. (This question was asked only of insurers who had not formally evaluated their preadmission review program. Thus, it may not be generalizable to the other insurers.) Concurrent and retrospective review of inpatient care were not seen to have this adverse effect, however.

Thirty-six of the group insurers practiced retrospective review of outpatient care, but only 13 had formally evaluated their program. Seven of the thirteen believed the program reduced total cost, four were undecided, and two reported higher total cost. The 23 firms that had not formally evaluated this program gave it more mixed reviews, however. Only six believed it was effective or somewhat effective in reducing outpatient cost and utilization. Eleven felt it had not been effective, and six gave other answers. Of the firms that believed the program was not effective, four felt that retrospective review resulted in higher outpatient cost and utilization. This is surprising, since the program is targeted toward outpatient care. It is possible that retrospective review of outpatient care produces some savings, but that these are outweighed by the costs of conducting the program.

**Figure A.4** Percentage of Individual Business Covered by Utilization Management Programs, 1988

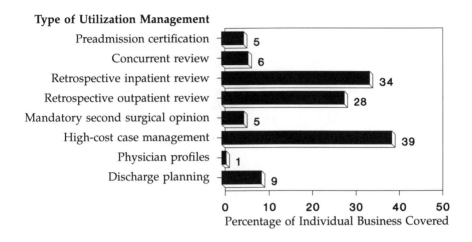

Type of Utilization Management

Source: HIAA Managed Care Survey, 1988.

*Other volume controls*

Preventing multiple physicians from billing for the same service, such as eliminating payments for an assistant surgeon, is the next most popular control after utilization review. Although 31 of the 132 companies practiced some form of this policy, only five companies had formally evaluated the effectiveness of their programs in this area. When asked for their overall impression, many respondents said they felt that preventing multiple billing had reduced cost and utilization outside the hospital.

Only 13 companies said they provided physician profiling and feedback in their commercial group health insurance. Companies attempting this form of control believed that it reduced total cost, but the sample was too small to place any confidence in the magnitude of estimated cost savings.

The survey did not ask about the use of clinical guidelines. Although it is tempting to equate physician profiling and feedback with the use of guidelines, it would be incorrect to do so. Profiling can be done without guidelines (the insurance company could simply collect profile data and send it to physicians). Similarly, guidelines do not require the carrier to keep physician profiles. Utilization review programs,

**Figure A.5**　Perceived Effectiveness of Utilization Management in Reducing Claims Costs in Group Business, 1988

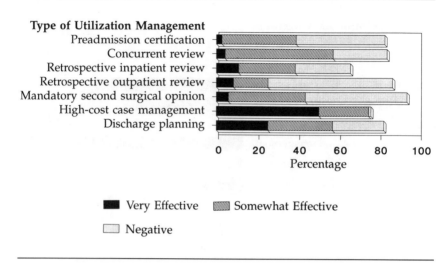

*Source:* HIAA Managed Care Survey, 1988.

for example, can use guidelines without keeping individual physician profiles.

Coding changes were not used extensively. Twenty-two companies reported implementing coding changes as a way to control physician services. Many of the respondents were unaware of procedure or coding changes, and when this type of volume and intensity control was explained to them, they were generally skeptical that it would control total cost and utilization. Others, when asked why they had not opted to change their coding to constrain outlays, responded, "Our company is not big enough," or "We just haven't done it," or "We lack the ability to do it correctly."

Finally, 15 companies reported bundling of physician services into broader categories than visits or procedures, such as single payment per episode of illness. The overall feeling toward bundling of services tended to be negative.

### Preferred provider organizations

Of the 123 firms surveyed, 72 had PPO arrangements. Unlike conventional insurance, PPOs do not typically use billed or usual charges to reimburse physicians. Forty-seven companies used fee schedules and 42

**Figure A.6**   Perceived Effectiveness of Utilization Management in
Reducing Claims Costs in Individual Business, 1988

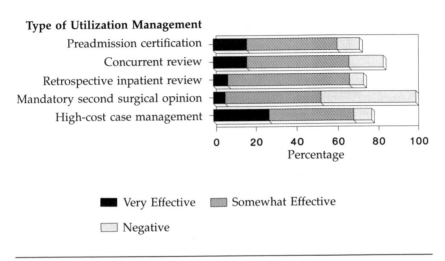

**Type of Utilization Management**

Preadmission certification

Concurrent review

Retrospective inpatient review

Mandatory second surgical opinion

High-cost case management

■ Very Effective    ▨ Somewhat Effective

☐ Negative

*Source:* HIAA Managed Care Survey, 1988.

used discounted charges. When more than one reimbursement method
was used, fee schedules were used most often. The types of physician
reimbursement that PPOs used are shown in Table A.3.

By volume of business, fee schedules and, to a lesser extent, discounted usual charges emerge as the most popular methods used by
insurer-sponsored PPOs for paying physicians (Figure A.7). The movement toward discounted usual charges was modest from 1986 to 1988.
Insurer-sponsored HMOs use capitation payment, which is the method
for paying the contracted physician group rather than the individual
physician, as their primary reimbursement method (Figure A.8).

Fifty-four of the 72 companies that have PPO arrangements responded to this question: "To the best of your knowledge, what percent
discount does the PPO receive from the preferred physicians?" The most
common answer, reported by 13 firms, was 15 percent. The mean answer
was 13.2 percent.

Firms were asked to rank the importance of several methods that
PPOs used to achieve savings. Utilization review received the highest
ranking by far. It was followed by discounts, channeling patients to cost-
effective providers, and provider reimbursement methods (Table A.4).
The importance given to utilization review is impressive, especially since
PPOs were receiving an average discount of 13.2 percent. Evidently, they

**Table A.3**  Methods Used by PPOs to Reimburse Physicians

| Method | Number of Firms Using | Number of Firms Not Using | Don't Know |
|---|---|---|---|
| Billed usual charges | 15 | 56 | 1 |
| Discounted usual charges | 42 | 29 | 1 |
| Fee schedule | 47 | 24 | 1 |
| Capitation | 5 | 66 | 1 |
| Other | 3 | 68 | 1 |

believed that UR reduced costs by more that 13.2 percent. To an extent, the importance given to "discounts" and "provider reimbursement methods" may reflect similar beliefs. Nevertheless, UR remains the most important cost-saving method, even considering the high ranks given to discounts and other provider reimbursement methods.

Next, insurers were asked about the utilization review programs conducted by their PPOs. All but two of the PPOs had a preadmission utilization review program. In 52 cases, UR was conducted by an automated system. Somewhat surprisingly, 30 of the 72 PPOs did not levy penalties on physicians or hospitals that refused to comply with utilization review. Of the 33 companies that mentioned some type of penalty, 13 used suspension or termination of the noncompliant provider, and 14 used a set dollar amount per episode. Forty-four PPOs penalized patients for failure to comply with the utilization review process. The most common penalties were increased deductibles (mentioned 16 times) and increased coinsurance (mentioned 12 times).

Fifty-one (71 percent) of the PPOs compiled and evaluated physician profiles, up from 40 percent in 1986. Profiles typically are compiled and evaluated by an automated procedure. Twenty-nine PPOs had a separate psychiatric utilization review program.

PPOs continue to devote less effort in selecting preferred physicians than they do in selecting preferred hospitals. Hospital privileges are the primary criterion (along with a catch-all "other" category) in selecting preferred physicians. About 60 percent of the PPOs identified a data source for selecting preferred physicians. The leading data source was insurer claims.

## Discussion

All Medicare and most private-sector health insurance carriers have utilization review programs, although Medicare carriers appear to focus more on reviewing the appropriateness of physician services than do

**Figure A.7** What Were the Primary Methods that Insurer-Sponsored PPOs Used to Reimburse Physicians in 1986 and 1988?

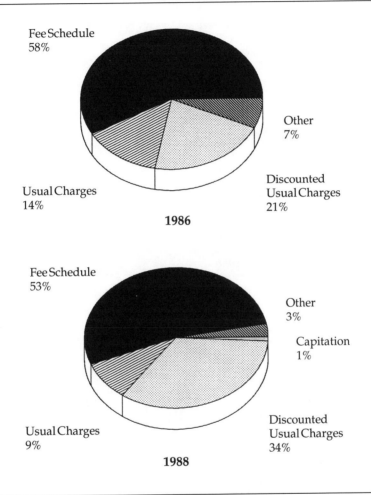

Fee Schedule
58%

Other
7%

Discounted
Usual Charges
21%

Usual Charges
14%

**1986**

Fee Schedule
53%

Other
3%

Capitation
1%

Discounted
Usual Charges
34%

Usual Charges
9%

**1988**

*Sources:* HIAA Managed Care Surveys, 1986 and 1988.

private carriers. This is partly because of the presence of mandated pre-payment screens for Medicare. Many Medicare carriers had these screens before they were mandated, however, and in some cases their preman-date screening guidelines were tighter than those implemented by Medi-care. Several mandated prepayment screens were cited frequently as ineffective, whereas other optional screens were suggested for inclusion in the list of mandated screens.

**Figure A.8**    How Did HMOs Use Capitation Payment for Paying
Physicians in 1986 and 1988?

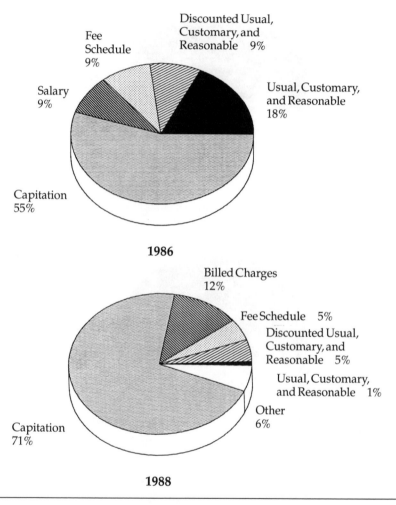

1986

1988

*Sources:* HIAA Managed Care Surveys, 1986 and 1988.

Medicare carriers suggested that new screens be introduced along
with programs to educate physicians about these screens. In general,
implementation issues are important and should not be ignored. On the
other hand, provider resistance to prepayment screens is not necessarily
a sign that they are ineffective.

**Table A.4**    Rank of Methods Used by PPOs to Achieve Savings

| | Rank | | | | |
|---|---|---|---|---|---|
| Method | 1 (most important) | 2 | 3 | 4 (least important) | Not Asked |
| Utilization review | 39 | 10 | 9 | 3 | 11 |
| Discount | 14 | 20 | 12 | 17 | 9 |
| Channeling patients to cost-effective providers | 9 | 19 | 15 | 20 | 9 |
| Provider reimbursement methods | 5 | 11 | 24 | 21 | 11 |

Medicare carriers operate vigorous postpayment review programs. In many cases, physicians are reviewed if their practice patterns are more than two standard deviations from the norm. However, the criteria for postpayment review are not uniform. Standards based on reviewing a prespecified number of physicians may be difficult to justify in detecting unusual practice patterns.

Private insurance carriers were found to operate inpatient utilization review programs that combine preadmission certification, concurrent review, and retrospective review of hospital inpatient care. The respondents estimated that inpatient utilization review reduces total cost by about 7 percent. Many believe that preadmission certification increases cost and utilization outside the hospital, however.

In managed fee-for-service programs, utilization review has been largely directed at reducing the use of inappropriate inpatient services. PPOs have made far less effort to select preferred physicians than to select hospitals, often using hospital staff privileges as the major screening criterion. HMOs have historically achieved their savings by reducing the number of hospital days.

Private carriers have been slow to initiate innovations in the area of physician payment. Out of 132 group insurers, all but eight still paid usual and customary charges. Only six respondents used "controlled" methods of paying physicians. Commercial insurers appear to place more emphasis on physician payment reform in their PPO arrangements, which frequently use discounted charges or fee schedules to pay physicians. The average discount was estimated to be about 13 percent, and this was exceeded in importance by the cost-saving effect of utilization review.

Perhaps the most significant result from our surveys is that neither public nor private carriers had taken an innovative approach to bundling physician services and collapsing the codes used for paying physicians. The private respondents generally were ignorant of this concept; most Medicare carriers thought that they had to recognize HCPCS codes for billing. Medicare carriers appear to be ahead of the private sector in using global fees for surgery, but otherwise they have not attempted to bundle physician services into broader reimbursement packages.

Physician education and feedback are used more extensively by Medicare carriers than by private insurers. This may be because they lead the private sector in postpayment review—the area where physician education programs are most likely to occur. Medicare carriers, in general, are sensitive to the need for physician education and information programs.

## Note

1. From *Medicare Carriers Manual*, Part 3—Claims Process (Washington, DC: U.S. GPO, 1988), 7–141.

# Index

# About the Authors

**Mark V. Pauly, Ph.D.,** is Bendheim Professor, professor and chairman of health care systems, professor of insurance and risk management, and professor of public policy and management at the University of Pennsylvania's Wharton School. He is also professor of economics in the School of Arts & Sciences and director of the Center for Research at Penn's Leonard Davis Institute of Health Economics. He is a member of the Institute of Medicine and an adjunct scholar of the American Enterprise Institute, and he has served on a number of technical advisory panels for groups such as the Advisory Council on Social Security, the Health Care Financing Administration's Division of National Cost Estimates, and the Congressional Budget Office. He is a member of the editorial boards of *Public Finance Quarterly, Health Services Research*, the *Journal of Risk and Uncertainty*, and the *Journal of Health Economics*. Dr. Pauly has published more than 100 journal articles and books in the fields of health economics, public finance, health insurance, and comparative health systems. He holds an M.A. from the University of Delaware and a Ph.D. from the University of Virginia.

**John M. Eisenberg, M.D., M.B.A.,** is the Anton and Margaret Fuisz Professor of Medicine and chairman and physician-in-chief in the Department of Medicine at Georgetown University's School of Medicine. He conducted the original research for this book while he was Sol Katz Professor and Chief of General Internal Medicine at the University of Pennsylvania's Medical Center (where earlier he completed his residency in internal medicine), professor of health care systems at Penn's Wharton School (where he took his M.B.A.), and senior fellow of the Leonard Davis Institute of Health Economics. Dr. Eisenberg is a member of the Physician Payment Review Commission and the Institute of Medicine, and he serves on the board of governors of the American Board of Internal Medicine. He is past president of the Association for Health Services Research and has served as president of the Society of General Internal Medicine, vice president of the Society for Medical Decision Making, and member of the board of regents of the American College of Physicians. Dr. Eisenberg's expertise in physician decision making and medical practice management, clinical economics, and medical education includes nearly 150 publications in the clinical medicine and health economics literature.

**Margaret Higgins Radany, M.P.P.,** was a research associate and project manager at the University of Pennsylvania's Leonard Davis Institute of Health Economics at the time the original research for this book was conducted. She holds a master's degree in public policy from Georgetown University and has research interests in technology assessment, medical practice patterns, and health care outcomes, in addition to physician payment. Her other publications, which reflect these interests, focus on the pricing or use of technology and the description of medical practice. Subsequent to her work at the University of Pennsylvania, she has been a research associate at the Institute for Health Policy Studies at the University of California at San Francisco.

**M. Haim Erder, Ph.D.,** is health economics scientist for The Upjohn Company where he conducts studies in pharmacoeconomics. Prior to joining Upjohn, Dr. Erder was senior research scholar for the Leonard Davis Institute of Health Economics where, in addition to work on the volume and intensity of physician services, he conducted studies in long-term care financing, adverse selection in multiple option group insurance, and costs of ambulatory surgery. Dr. Erder's other publications and research interests are in the areas of emergency medical care and biotechnology. He holds a Ph.D. in public policy from the University of Pennsylvania's Wharton School.

**Roger Feldman, Ph.D.,** is professor of health services research and policy and professor of economics at the University of Minnesota. He serves as director of the Health Care Financing Research Center, a consortium of more than 50 scholars from the University of Minnesota, the University of Pennsylvania, and Mathematica Policy Research, Inc., under which the original grant for this work was funded. Dr. Feldman has served as a senior staff economist for the President's Council of Economic Advisors and a member of the expert panel on health care costs for the Congressional Budget Office. In addition, he serves on numerous grant review panels for such organizations as the Health Care Financing Administration, the Agency for Health Care Policy and Research, and the National

Science Foundation. He sits on the editorial boards of *Health Services Research, Inquiry,* and the *Quarterly Review of Economics and Business.* Dr. Feldman's Ph.D. in economics is from the University of Rochester.

**J. Sanford Schwartz, M.D.,** is associate professor of medicine at the University of Pennsylvania's School of Medicine, associate professor of health care systems and the Robert D. Eilers Associate Professor of Health Care Management and Economics at The Wharton School, and executive director of Penn's Leonard Davis Institute of Health Economics. He is past president and member of the board of trustees of the American Federation for Clinical Research, a member of the Council of Academic Societies of the Association of American Medical Colleges, chair of the Technology Assessment Committee of the Society for General Internal Medicine, and former president of the Society for Medical Decision Making. In addition, he serves on the editorial board of the *Journal of General Internal Medicine.* Dr. Schwartz received his M.D. from the University of Pennsylvania's School of Medicine, where he also was a Robert Wood Johnson Foundation Clinical Scholar. His work in the evaluation of medical practices and medical decision making is widely published and addresses topics such as the evaluation of trade-offs among cost, quality, and outcomes and ways to optimize the value of clinical information.